Biochemistry Workbook for Medical Students

A Classroom Companion

As per the latest NMC Guidelines | Competency Based Medical Education (CBME) Curriculum under Graduate Medical Education Regulation

Biochemistry Workbook
for Medical Students
A Classroom Companion

As per the latest NMC Guidelines | Competency Based Medical Education (CBME) Curriculum under Graduate Medical Education Regulation

Poonam Agrawal MBBS, MD, FIMSA, ACME

Professor and Head
Department of Biochemistry
Santosh Medical College
Santosh Deemed to be University
Ghaziabad, UP

former Professor and Head
Department of Biochemistry
Dr Baba Saheb Ambedkar Medical College and Hospital
New Delhi

CBSPD

CBS Publishers & Distributors Pvt Ltd

New Delhi • Bengaluru • Chennai • Kochi • Kolkata • Lucknow • Mumbai
Hyderabad • Jharkhand • Nagpur • Patna • Pune • Uttarakhand

Disclaimer

Science and technology are constantly changing fields. New research and experience broaden the scope of information and knowledge. The author has tried her best in giving information available to her while preparing the material for this book. Although all efforts have been made to ensure optimum accuracy of the material, yet it is quite possible some errors might have been left uncorrected. The publisher, the printer and the author will not be held responsible for any inadvertent errors or inaccuracies.

Biochemistry
Workbook
for Medical Students
A Classroom Companion

ISBN: 978-93-5466-824-1

First Edition: 2025

Published by Satish Kumar Jain and produced by Varun Jain for

CBS Publishers & Distributors Pvt Ltd

4819/XI Prahlad Street, 24 Ansari Road, Daryaganj, New Delhi 110 002, India.
Ph: 011-23289259, 23266838 Website: www.cbspd.com
e-mail: delhi@cbspd.com

Corporate Office: 204 FIE, Industrial Area, Patparganj, Delhi 110 092, India
Ph: 011-4934 4934 Fax: 011-4934 4935 e-mail: publishing@cbspd.com; publicity@cbspd.com

Branches

- **Bengaluru:** Seema House 2975, 17th Cross, K.R. Road, Banasankari 2nd Stage, Bengaluru 560 070, Karnataka, India
  Ph: +91-80-26771678/79 Fax: +91-80-26771680 e-mail: bangalore@cbspd.com
- **Chennai:** 7, Subbaraya Street, Shenoy Nagar, Chennai 600 030, Tamil Nadu, India
  Ph: +91-44-26680620, 26681266 Fax: +91-44-42032115 e-mail: chennai@cbspd.com
- **Kochi:** 42/1325, 36, Power House Road, Opposite KSEB, Ernakulam 682 018 Kochi, Kerala, India
  Ph: +91-484-4059061-65, 67 Fax: +91-484-4059065 e-mail: kochi@cbspd.com
- **Kolkata:** 147, Hind Ceramics Compound, 1st Floor, Nilgunj Road, Belghoria, Kolkata 700 056, West Bengal, India
  Ph: +91-33-25633055/56 e-mail: kolkata@cbspd.com
- **Lucknow:** Basement, Khushnuma Complex, 7-Meerabai Marg (Behind Jawahar Bhawan), Lucknow-226 001, Uttar Pradesh, India
  Ph: +910522-4000032 e-mail: tiwari.lucknow@cbspd.com
- **Mumbai:** PWD Shed, Gala No. 25/26, Ramchandra Bhatt Marg, Next to JJ Hospital Gate No. 2, Opp Union Bank of India, Noorbaug, Mumbai-400009, Maharashtra, India
  Ph: +91-22-66661880/89 e-mail: mumbai@cbspd.com

Representatives

- **Hyderabad** 0-9885175004
- **Patna** 0-9334159340
- **Jharkhand** 0-9811541605
- **Pune** 0-9664372571
- **Nagpur** 0-8692091830
- **Uttarakhand** 0-9716462459

Printed at: Shri Prints & Sales, Delhi, India

to

My beloved students who strive hard to become the healer

Preface

Learning biochemistry in medical school always pose a challenge, largely due to complexity of metabolic pathways and vast information which students need to remember before it can be applied in actual practice.

In almost two decades of my teaching experience, I have perceived that medical students consider this subject difficult and struggle to remember various factual information for longer duration. Even during classroom teaching students often loose track and tend to skip many crucial information shared by their teachers, mainly because of lack of any handy resource material which might help them to be on track and make learning more directional and easier.

To help students to overcome these learning barriers, I have developed this *Biochemistry Workbook for Medical Students: A Classroom Companion* which has all the important pathways, flowcharts, and diagrams arranged in sequential manner along with the key concepts of the topic. I have taken special interest in highlighting the clinical and applied aspects of the topic so that the subject is relevant to medical students and retention and recall rate is higher.

Additionally, if used consistently this module will prove to be a crisp, complete and diagrammatic resource material with self-written golden key notes, which not only will give confidence to the learner but also will turn out to be a ready resource material which can be quickly revised at a very short notice before the examination.

My suggestion to make best use of this workbook is to carry it everyday to the classroom and follow it along with the classroom teaching and jot down important points shared by the teacher in the workbook itself in space provided.

I strongly believe that this workbook will turn out to be a boon for medical students for learning biochemistry. Wishing you very best for your journey towards excellence!!

Poonam Agrawal
Connect with me@
drpoonam24agrawal@yahoo.com

Acknowledgments

Gratitude to that Supreme Power for all the kindness he showers on me each day. I am indebted to many for this work. First of all, I acknowledge contribution of my students, who always inspire me to learn more and share more. Their faith in me gives me the actual strength to work harder and do innovations in medical education to make learning easy and relevant.

I am thankful for the acceptability of views and support of Mr SK Jain (CMD) and Mr Varun Jain (Director), CBS Publishers & Distributors Pvt Ltd. I am obliged for continuous support from Mr YN Arjuna (Senior Vice-President—Publishing, Editorial and Publicity); and his entire team, especially Mrs Ritu Chawla (AGM—Production), Ananda Mohanty (Proofreader) Mrs Ritu Tiwari (InDesign Operator), Mr Manish Raj (Graphic Designer). I appreciate the entire team of CBS Publishers & Distributors in the shaping of this book.

My husband Dr Mohit Agarwal, my daughter Ms Agrima, my parents Dr Shri Prakash Agarwal, Mrs Manu Agarwal, Mr Ram Baboo Agarwal, Late Smt Adesh Agarwal who always support me with their unconditional love and encourage me to make best use of my time and contribute to the society in whatever manner I can.

My pet dear Peenu (Mr Peanut) deserve special mention, who share special bond with me and my family.

Poonam Agrawal

Contents

Section F: DNA Replication, Transcription, Translation and Gene Regulation

Section G: Genetic Technologies

Section H: Heme

Section I: Enzyme

Section J: Miscellaneous

Section A
Carbohydrates and their Metabolism

1

Carbohydrate Chemistry

1. WHAT IS CARBOHYDRATE?/DEFINE CARBOHYDRATES

Carbohydrates are aldehyde or keto-derivatives of polyhydroxy alcohols or substances which yield such compounds on hydrolysis.

2. CLASSIFICATION OF CARBOHYDRATES

Carbohydrates are classified based on a number of individual monosaccharide units derived from the complete hydrolysis of the carbohydrate compound.

Accordingly, they are classified into the following four major groups:

- Monosaccharides
- Disaccharides
- Oligosaccharides
- Polysaccharides

Key Notes

Table 1.1: Monosaccharides

General formula	Aldosugar	Ketosugar
Triose	Glyceraldehyde or Glycerose	Dihydroxyacetone
Tetrose	Erythrose	Erythrulose
Pentose	Ribose (Xylose, Arabinose)	Ribulose, Xylulose
Hexose	Glucose, Galactose, Mannose	Fructose
Heptose	Glucoheptose	Sedoheptulose
Nanose	Sialic acid (NANA)	—

Table 1.2: List of disaccharides

Disaccharides	Reducing (R) or nonreducing (NR)	Individual monosaccharide units	Bonds
Sucrose α-D-glucopyranosyl β-D-fructofuranoside	Nonreducing	Glucose + Fructose	α-1, β-2
Trehalose	Nonreducing	Glucose + Glucose	α-1,1-glycosidic
Maltose	Reducing	Glucose + Glucose	α-1,4-glycosidic
Isomaltose	Reducing	Glucose + Glucose	α-1,6-glycosidic
Lactose	Reducing	Glucose + Galactose	β-1,4-glycosidic
Lactulose	Reducing	Fructose + Galactose	β-1,4-glycosidic

Key Notes

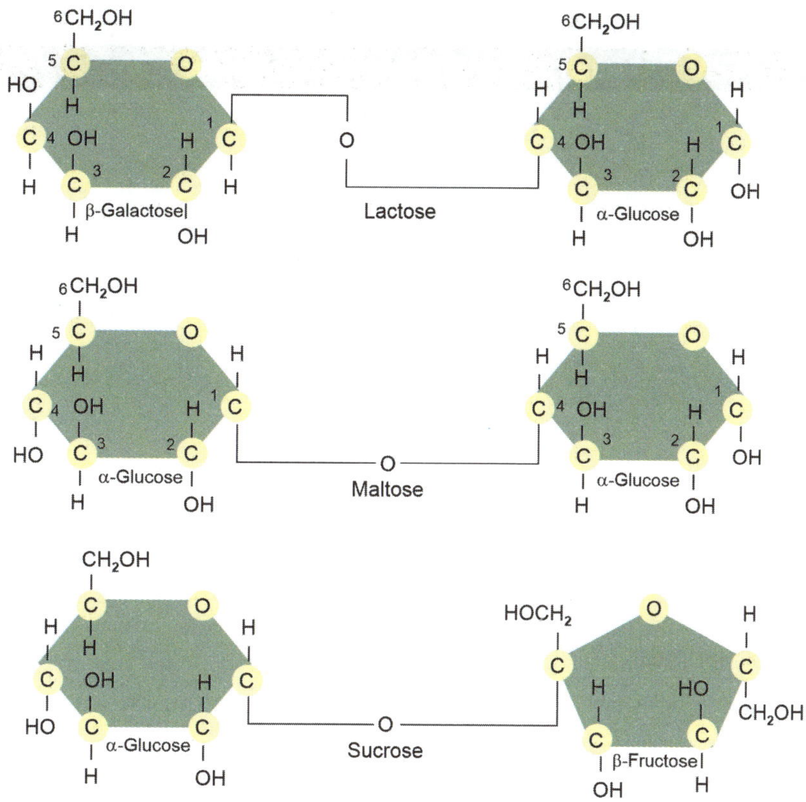

Fig. 1.1: Disaccharides

Oligosaccharides

They have 3–10 residues of monosaccharide linked together
Examples are: Limit dextrin, maltotriose

Polysaccharides

They have more than ten monosaccharide residues attached. These monosaccharides may be the same or different, accordingly, they are known as homopolysaccharides or heteropolysaccharides.

Key Notes

Homopolysaccharides

Table 1.3: List of homopolysaccharides		
Homopolysaccharides	**Units of monosaccharides**	**Bonds**
Starch	Glucose	α-1,4- and α-1,6-glycosidic bond
Glycogen	Glucose	α-1,4- and α-1,6-glycosidic bond
Cellulose	Glucose	β-1,4-glycosidic bond
Inulin	Fructose	β-1,2-glycosidic bond
Dextran	Glucose	α-1,6-glycosidic bond α-1,4-glycosidic bond α-1,3-glycosidic bond
Chitin	N-acetyl-D-glucosamine [NAG]	β-1,4-glycosidic bond

Heteropolysaccharides

Agar, agarose, pectin, gum, blood group antigen, and mucopolysaccharides are examples of heteropolysaccharides (HPS). MPS are also known as glycosaminoglycans (GAG).

3. STEREOISOMERS OF CARBOHYDRATE

Compounds having the same molecular formula but different structure formulas are known as structural isomers/ stereoisomers of each other.

A. Aldo–keto isomer

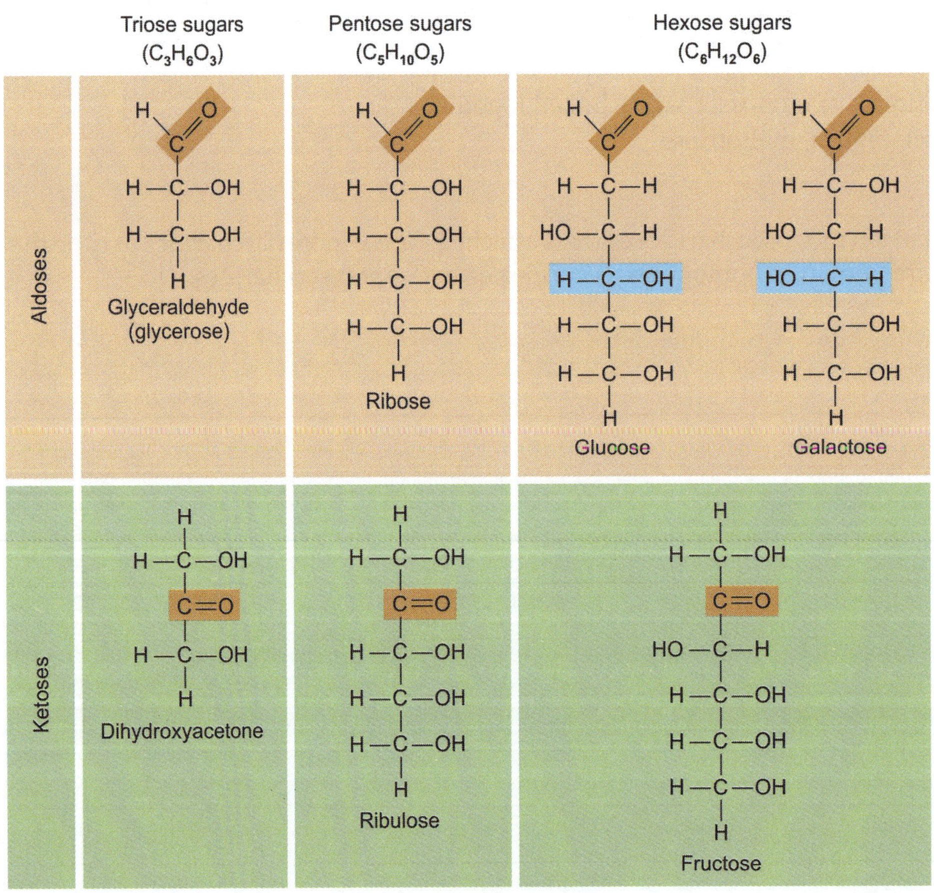

Fig. 1.2: Aldo–keto isomers

B. Epimers

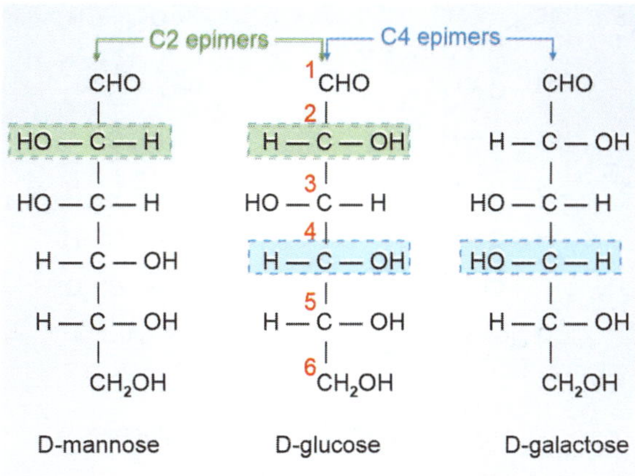

Fig. 1.3: C2 and C4 epimers of glucose

C. Pyranose–furanose type of isomers

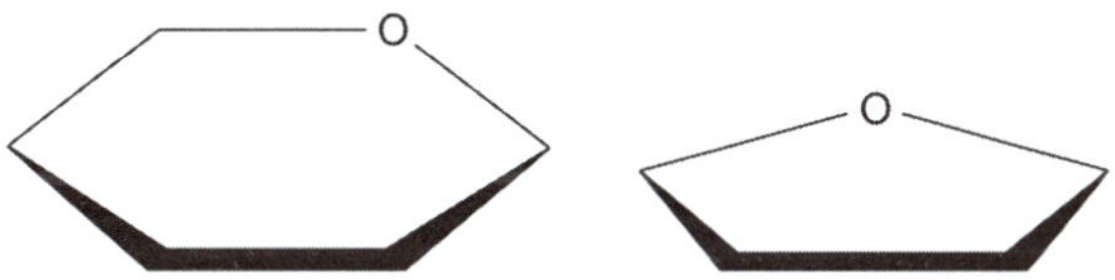

Fig. 1.4: Pyranose and furanose rings

D. Anomers (alpha and beta)

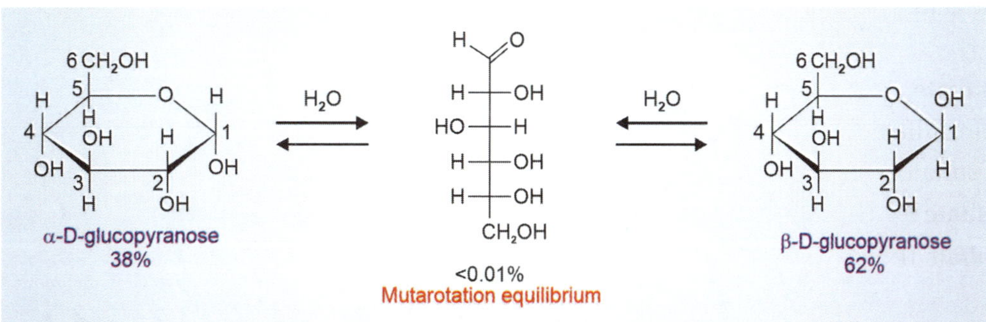

Fig. 1.5: Mutarotation equilibrium (in glucose)

E. D and L isomers [enantiomer]

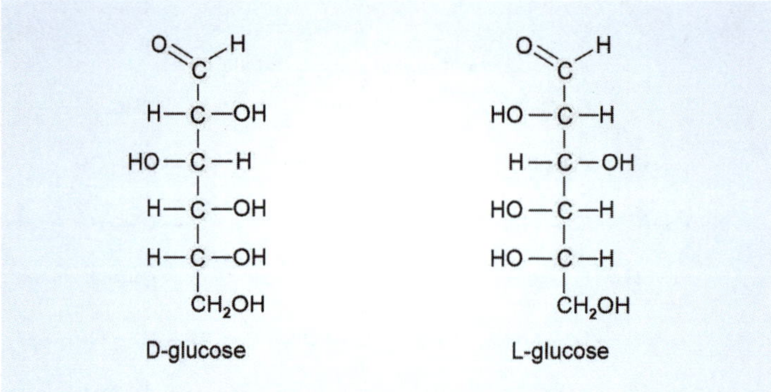

Fig. 1.6: D and L isomers of glucose

4. CLINICAL CORRELATION

Lactose intolerance

a. Enzyme deficiency: Lactase
b. Clinical presentation: Abdominal discomfort, bloating, cramps, diarrhea on consumption of milk and dairy products
c. Food to avoid: Milk and dairy products

5. CLINICAL UTILITY

a. Lactulose: Being used to induce osmotic diarrhea
b. Sucralose: Used as artificial sweetener

6. MUCOPOLYSACCHARIDES

Characteristics

- Made up of repeating units of amino sugar and uronic acid
- Most of them are highly sulfated (the exception is hyaluronic acid, which is not sulfated)
- They are negatively charged
- They are hygroscopic

Examples of mucopolysaccharides are

1. Hyaluronic acid
2. Heparin
3. Heparan sulfate
4. Chondroitin sulfate
5. Dermatan sulfate
6. Keratan sulfate I
7. Keratan sulfate II

Key Notes

2

Glucose Oxidation

Key concept of glucose oxidation
Main purpose of glucose oxidation is production of ATP.

Aerobic glucose oxidation comprises 3 stages

- Aerobic glycolysis
- PDH complex activity
- TCA cycle

Anaerobic glucose oxidation comprises only 1 stage

- Anaerobic glycolysis

GLYCOLYSIS

Also called the Embden Meyerhof pathway

Both aerobic and anaerobic glycolysis is cytosolic pathway
End product of aerobic glycolysis: Pyruvate
End product of anaerobic glycolysis: Lactate

ATP Production

- Aerobic glycolysis: Total 9, Net 7
- Anaerobic glycolysis: Total 4, Net 2
- PDH complex: 2.5 ATP from 1 pyruvate
- TCA cycle: 10 ATP from 1 acetyl-CoA

Key Notes

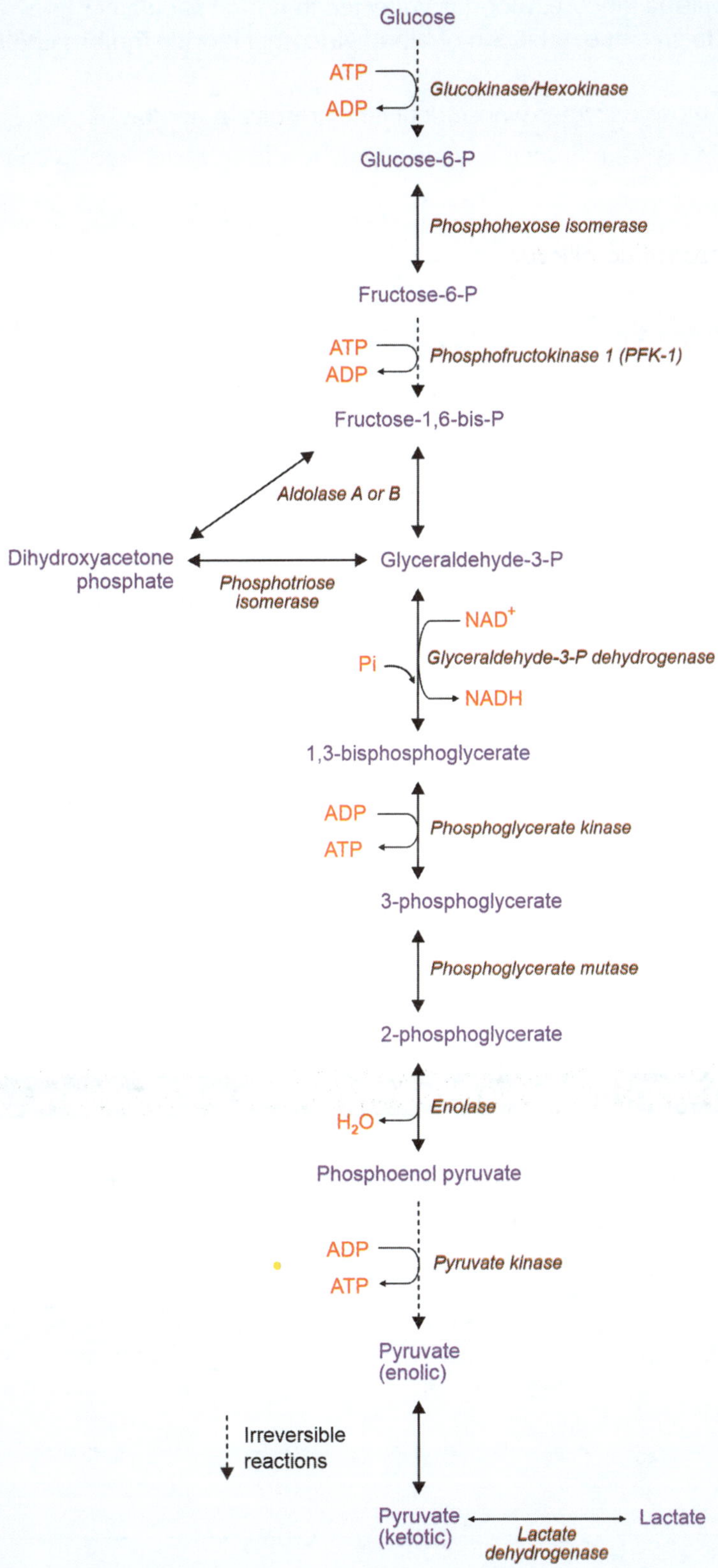

Fig. 2.1: Steps of glycolysis

Clinical Correlation

- For estimation of blood/plasma glucose, blood is collected in uoride vacutainer (grey cap) to prevent glycolysis in the collected blood as to give true reflection of blood glucose. Fluoride inhibits enolase enzyme and prevents glycolysis.
- Pyruvate kinase is one of those enzymes whose deficiency results in hemolysis
- *Crabtree effect:* Excess glycolysis in limited oxygen supply results in anaerobic glycolysis and hence lactic acid production.

Rate-limiting Step: PFK-1 (Phosphofructokinase 1)

1. Regulation of PFK-1

- Phosphofructokinase 1 (PFK-1) is a major regulatory enzyme of glycolysis.
- Phosphofructokinase 1 is an allosteric enzyme which has got its positive and negative allosteric factors.

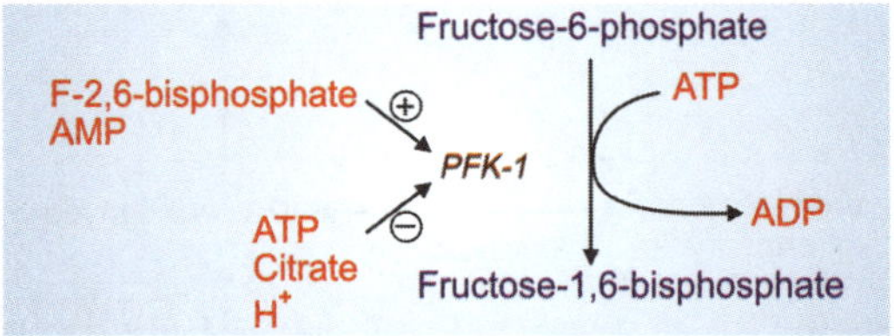

Fig. 2.2: Positive and negative allosteric modifiers of phosphofructokinase enzyme

Key point for PFK-1

Positive factors for PFK-1

- Fructose 2,6-bisphosphate 5′AMP

Negative factors for PFK-1

- ATP
- Citrate
- Protons

Table 2.1: Differences between hexokinase and glucokinase

	Hexokinase	Glucokinase
Site	All tissues except liver	Only in liver, β-cell of pancreas
Substrate	Glucose, fructose or galactose	Only glucose
Induction	Noninducible	Inducible
K_m for glucose	Low (0.05 mmol/L or 0.9 mg/dl)	High (10 mmol/L or 180 mg/dl)
Inhibition by glucose-6-phosphate	Inhibited	Not inhibited
Effect of feeding and insulin	No change in activity	Increased activity as well as rate of synthesis

Key Notes

Rapoport-Luebering Shunt (RL Shunt)

Key concepts for Rapoport-Luebering shunt

- RL shunt occurs in mature RBC for the purpose of production of 2,3-bisphosphoglycerate
- 2,3-bisphosphoglycerate helps in release of oxygen from the hemogobin, which facilitates delivery of oxygen to the tissues.
- Two key enzymes of Rapoport-Luebering shunt are:
  a. 1,3-bisphosphoglycerate mutase
  b. 2,3-bisphosphoglycerate phosphatase

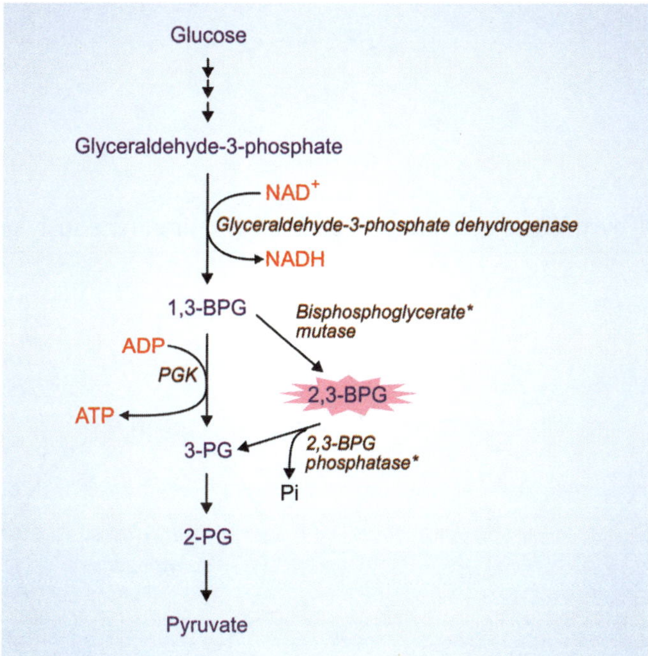

(*BPG mutase and BPG phosphatase are bifunctional enzymes which means one polypeptide has two catalytic domains)

Fig. 2.3: Rapoport-Luebering cycle (RL shunt)

Key Notes

PDH COMPLEX

Key concept of PDH complex

- Pyruvate is oxidatively decarboxylated to produce acetyl-CoA.

Enzymes of PDH complex

There are three enzymes in PDH complex which act in a sequential manner with the help of various coenzymes.

a. Pyruvate dehydrogenase (E1)

b. Dihydrolipoyl transacetylase (E2)

c. Dihydrolipoyl dehydrogenase (E3)

Coenzymes of PDH complex

- Thiamine pyrophosphate (TPP)
- Lipoate
- CoA-SH (coenzyme A-SH)
- FAD
- NAD

Energetics

- 1 NADH is produced when 1 pyruvate is converted to acetyl-CoA, simultaneously generating 2.5 ATP

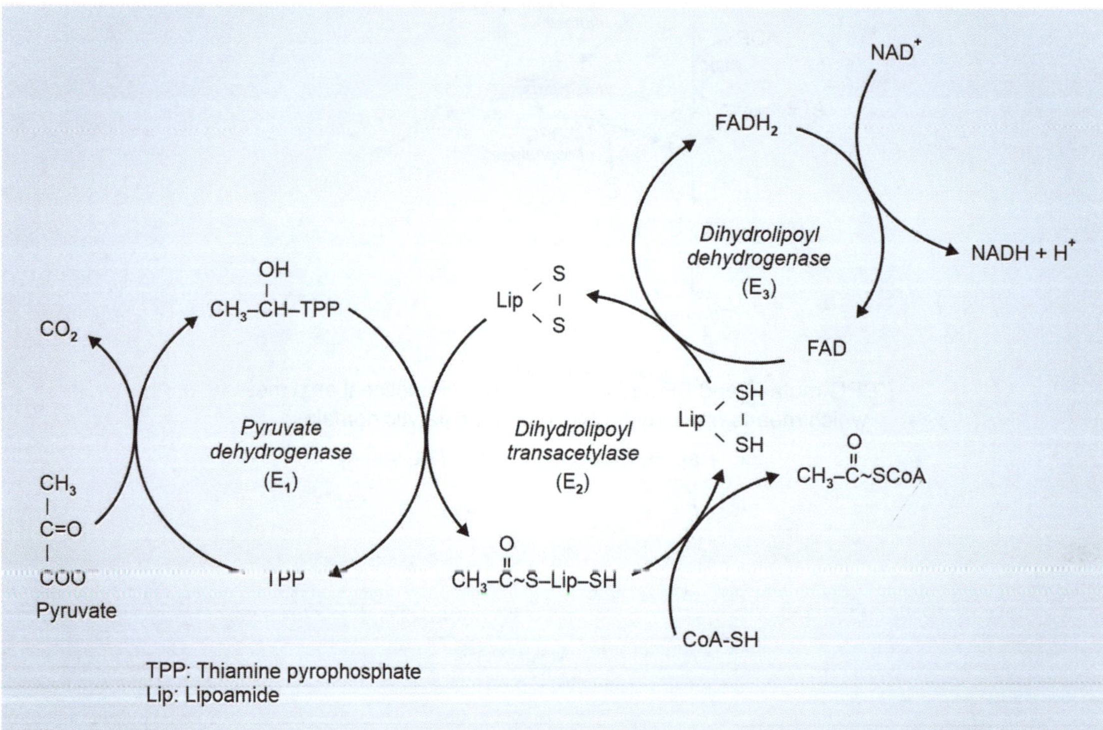

Fig. 2.4: PDH complex

Clinical Correlation

- In deficiency of vitamin B_1 or in case of mutation of any of the enzyme of PDH complex, lactic acidosis results due to diversion of pyruvate to lactate by LDH enzyme.
- Babies belonging to low socio-economic strata often present with features of B_1 deficiency (beriberi) where lactic acidosis is an important finding.

CITRIC ACID CYCLE (KREBS' CYCLE OR TCA CYCLE)

Key concepts

- ***TCA cycle:*** It is a series of enzyme catalyzed reactions that form a common pathway for final oxidation of acetyl-CoA coming from all metabolic fuels (carbohydrate, free fatty acids, ketone bodies and amino acids).
- ***Location:*** All the enzymes of TCA cycle (except succinate dehydrogenase) is dispersed in mitochondrial matrix. Succinate dehydrogenase is found at inner mitochondrial membrane.
- ***Bioenergetics:*** One molecule of acetyl-CoA produces 10 ATPs in a complete turn of citric acid cycle.

  TCA cycle is an amphibolic pathway which has role to play in catabolism of acetyl-CoA and various anabolic pathways of system.

Key Notes

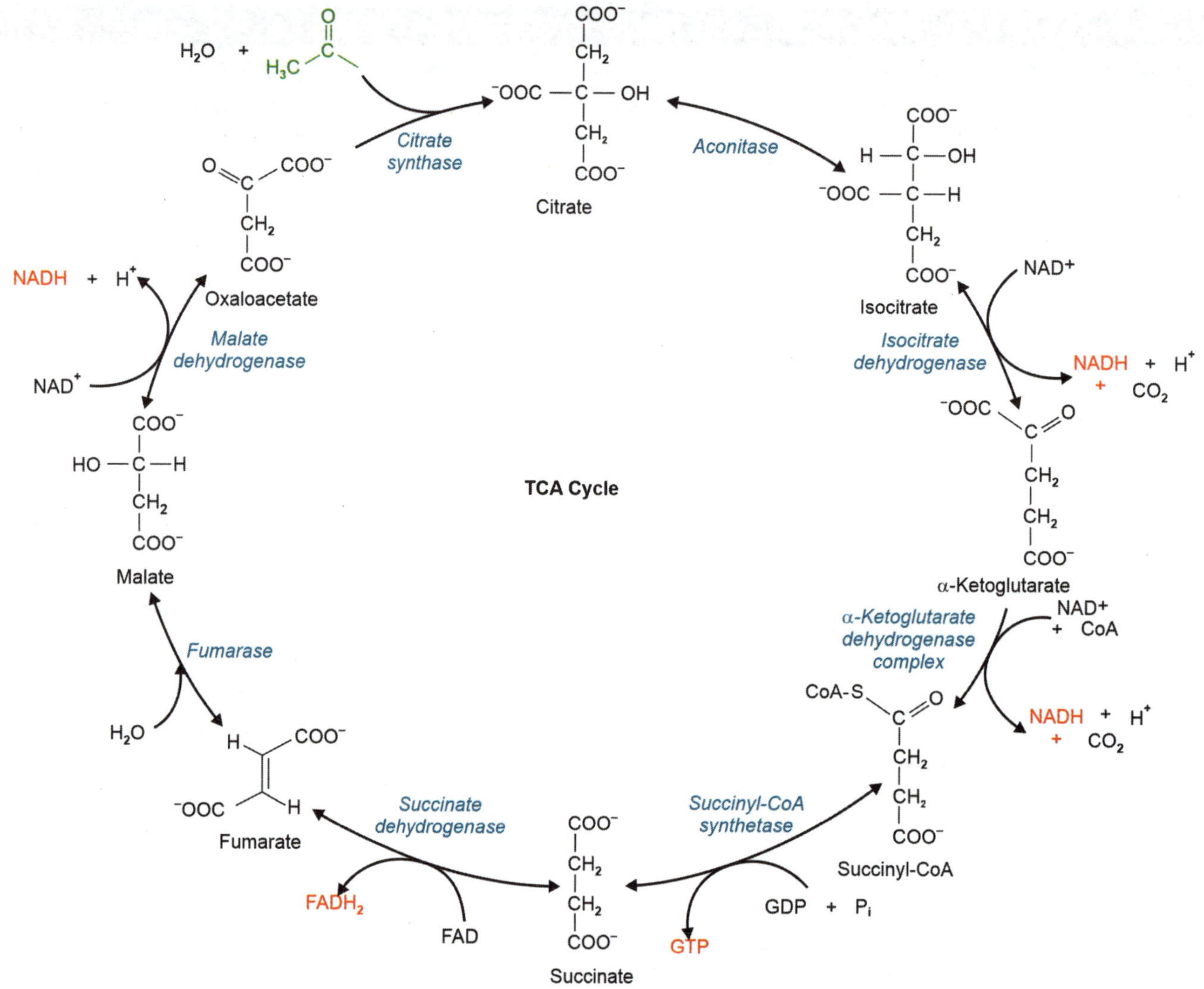

Fig. 2.5: TCA cycle

Key Notes

3

Gluconeogenesis

What is gluconeogenesis?

This is the process of formation of glucose from noncarbohydrate substances.

Substrate of gluconeogenesis

- *Glucogenic amino acid*
- *Lactate*
- *Pyruvate*
- *Propionate*
- *Glycerol*
- *Fumaric acid.*

Key concept for the process of gluconeogenesis

Reversible steps of the glycolysis are used in reverse direction and irreversible steps of glycolysis (pyruvate kinase, phosphofructokinase, glucokinase) are bypassed by exclusive reactions of gluconeogenesis.

Key Notes

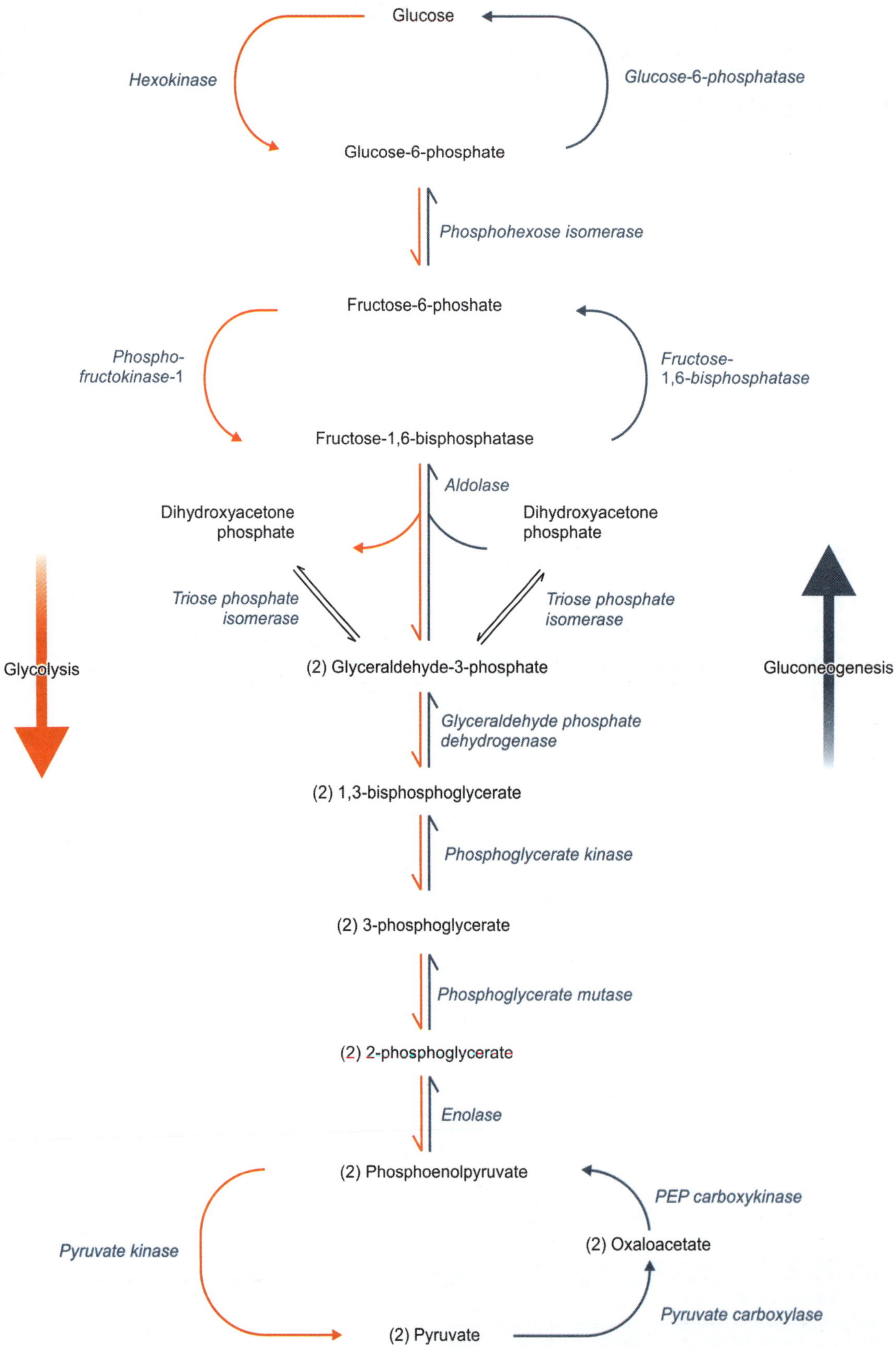

Fig. 3.1: Steps of glycolysis and gluconeogenesis

The above diagram shows how the reversible steps of glycolysis are used in a reverse direction and how irreversible steps of glycolysis are bypassed by new reactions during gluconeogenesis.

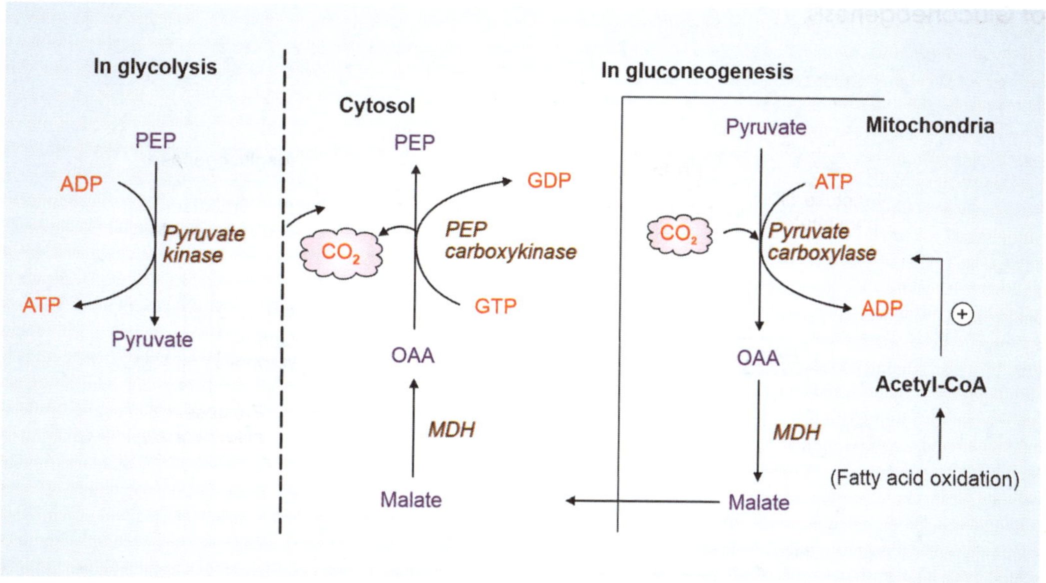

Fig. 3.2: Reversal of pyruvate kinase reaction

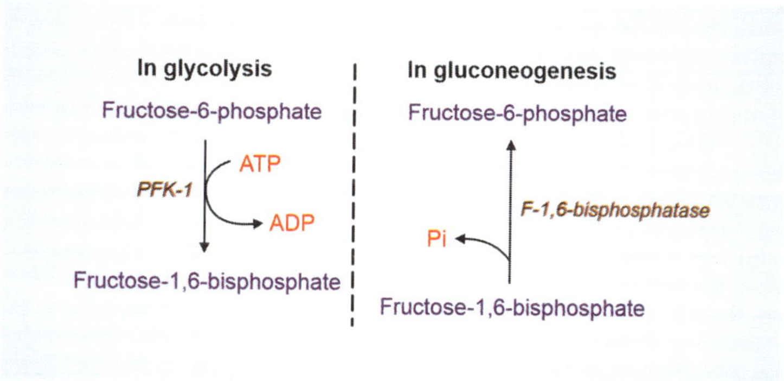

Fig. 3.3: Reversal of PFK-1 reaction

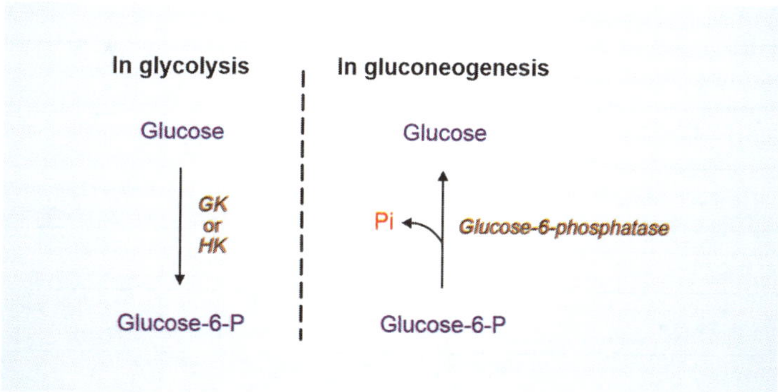

Fig. 3.4: Reversal of glucokinase/hexokinase reaction

Regulation of Gluconeogenesis

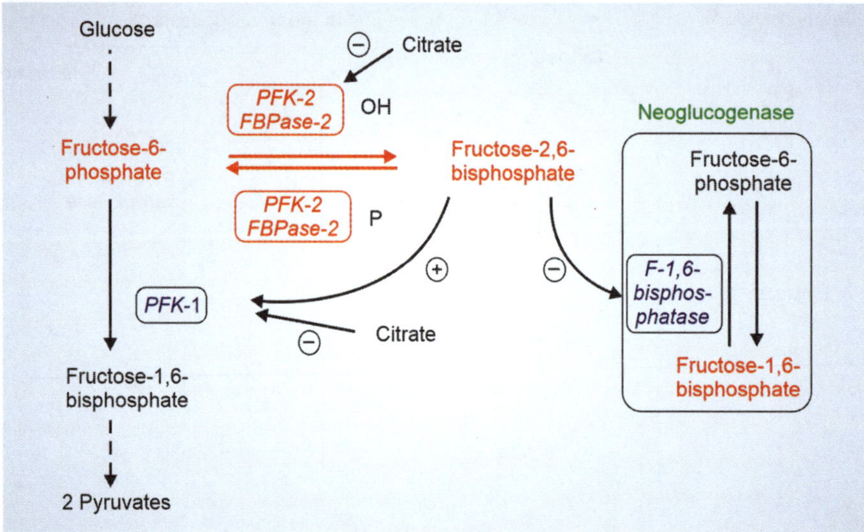

Fig. 3.5: Simultaneous regulation of PFK-1 and F-1,6-bisphosphatase by F-2,6-bisphosphate

Key Notes

CORI CYCLE

Key concept for Cori cycle

- Cori cycle is also known as glucose–lactate cycle.
- Anaerobic glycolysis in skeletal muscle during exercise and gluconeogenesis in liver constitute Cori cycle.
- During prolonged exercise muscle pain is due to accumulation of lactate, which gets diffused to blood on resting.

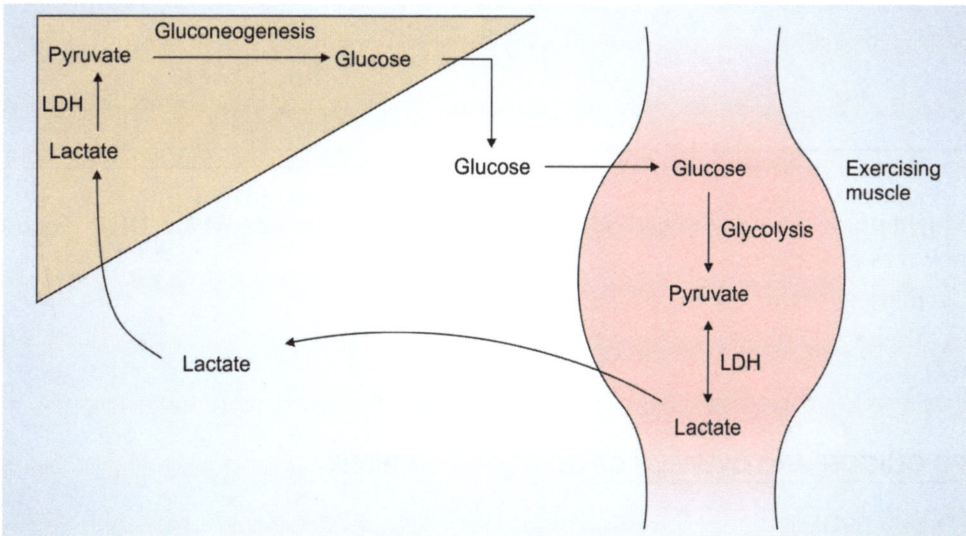

Fig. 3.6: Cori cycle (glucose–lactate cycle)

Key Notes

4

Glycogen Metabolism

GLYCOGENESIS

Key concepts

- Synthesis of highly branched polymer of glucose in a multistep process, where UDP glucose is the donor of glucose is known as glycogenesis.
- Organs involved in the process of glycogen metabolism
  - *Liver*
  - *Skeletal muscle*

SYNTHESIS OF UPD GLUCOSE AND OVERVIEW OF GLYCOGEN SYNTHESIS

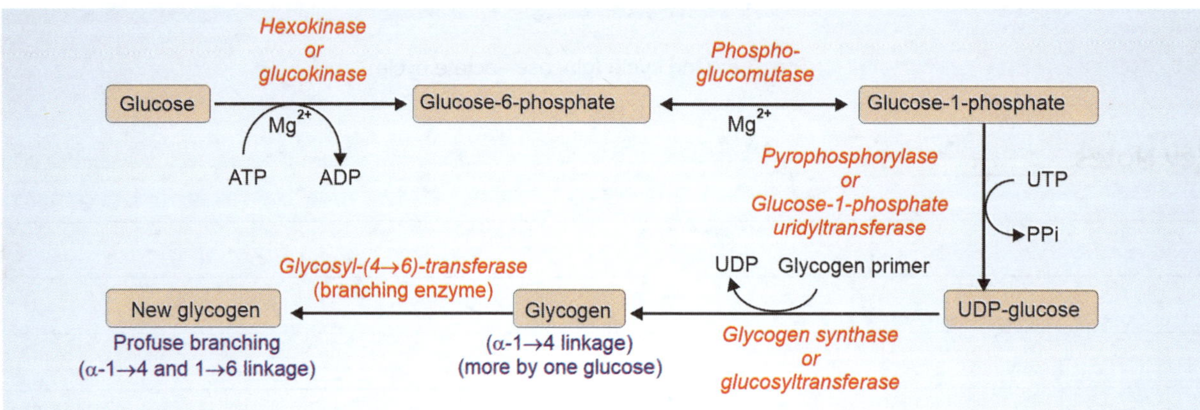

Fig. 4.1: Mechanism of glycogenesis

Key Notes

ACTION OF GLYCOGEN SYNTHASE AND BRANCHING ENZYME DURING GLYCOGENESIS

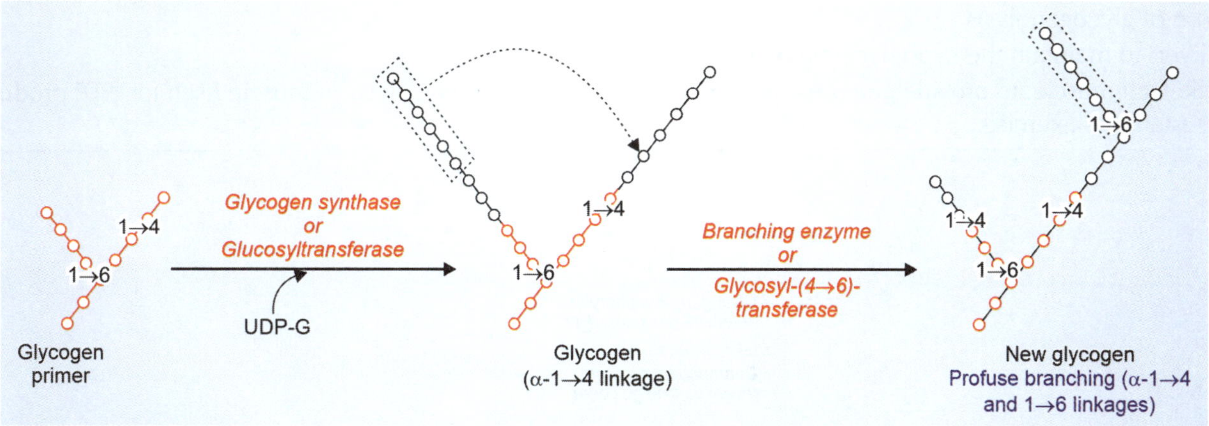

Fig. 4.2: Mechanism of glycogenesis

Key Notes

GLYCOGENOLYSIS

Key concepts

Purpose of glycogenolysis

- In liver: to maintain the hypoglycemia by releasing free glucose.
- In skeletal muscle: to provide glucose 6 phosphate which is used in glycolysis in muscle itself for ATP production to sustain the exercise.

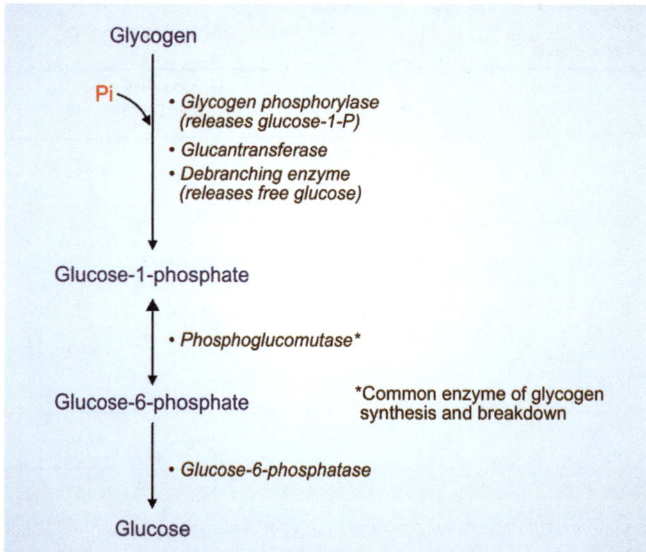

Fig. 4.3: Glycogen degradation (glycogenolysis)

Key Notes

Clinical Correlation

Glycogen Storage Diseases

Table 4.1: Glycogen storage disorders

Glyco-genesis	Name	Cause of disorder	Characteristics
Type 0	—	Glycogen synthase	Hypoglycemia, hyperketonemia, early death
Type Ia	Von Gierke disease	Deficiency of glucose-6-phosphatase	Hypoglycemia, lactic acidemia, ketosis, hyperlipemia
Type Ib	—	Endoplasmic reticulum glucose-6-phosphate transporter	As type Ia; neutropenia and impaired neutrophil function leading to recurrent infections
Type II*	Pompe disease	Deficiency of lysosomal α-1,4 and α-1,6-glucosidase	Fatal, accumulation of glycogen in lysosomes, skeletal and cardiac muscle involved, liver spared
Type IIIa	Cori/Forbes disease/ Limit dextrinosis	Absence of debranching enzyme in muscle and liver	Accumulation of characteristic branched polysaccharide in both
Type IIIb	Limit dextrinosis	Liver debranching enzyme is deficient	Accumulation of characteristic branched polysaccharide in liver alone
Type IV	Andersen disease, amylopectinosis	Absence of branching enzyme	Death due to cardiac or liver failure in the first year of life
Type V*	McArdle syndrome	Absence of muscle phosphorylase	Diminished exercise tolerance; muscles have abnormally high glycogen content
Type VI	Hers disease	Deficiency of liver (hepatic)	High glycogen content in liver, tendency towards hypoglycemia
Type VII*	Tarui's disease	Deficiency of muscle and RBC phospho-fructokinase	As in type V
Type VIII	—	Liver phosphorylase kinase	Hepatomegaly
Type IX	—	Liver and muscle phosphorylase kinase	Hepatomegaly
Type X	—	cAMP-dependent protein kinase A	Hepatomegaly
Type XI	Fanconi-Bickel disease	GLUT-2 in liver is affected	—

*Liver spared in: GSD type II, V, VII; muscle spared in: GSD type 0, Ia, Ib, IIIb, VI, VIII, IX, X

Key Notes

5

Galactose Metabolism

GALACTOSE METABOLISM

Key concepts

- Metabolism of galactose occurs only in the liver
- Galactokinase, galactose-1-phosphate uridyl transferase, 4-epimerase are the exclusive enzyme for galactose metabolism
- Any metabolic error in galactose metabolism results in increased level of galactose in the plasma which is excreted in the urine (galactosuria). Benedict's test will be positive in urine as galactose is the reducing sugar.

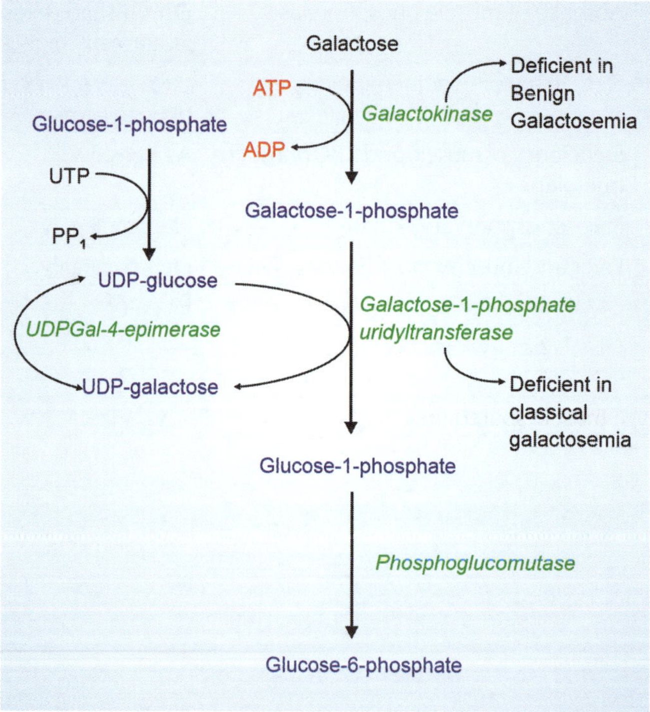

Fig. 5.1: Galactose metabolism

Key Notes

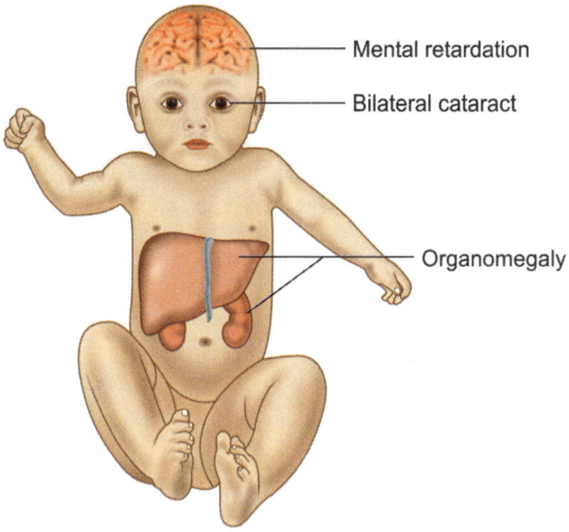

Fig. 5.2: A child with galactosemia

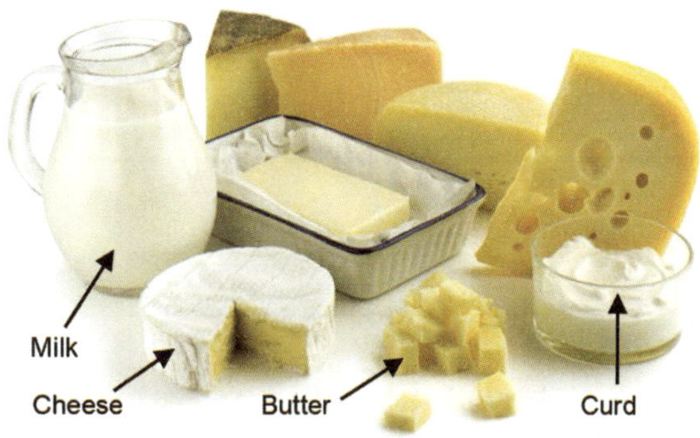

Fig. 5.3: Lactose-containing diet should be avoided in galactosemia

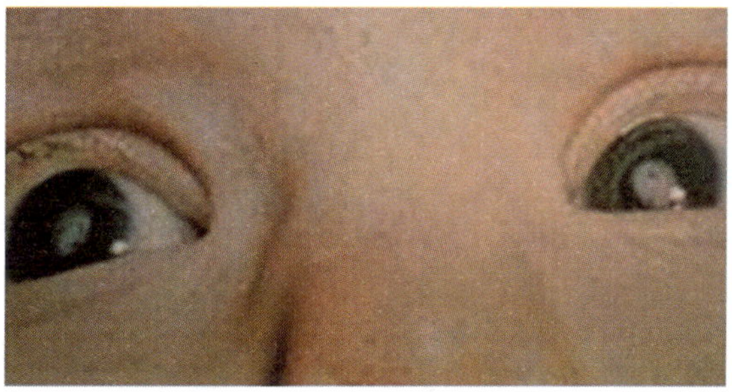

Fig. 5.4: Bilateral cataract in galactosemia

Clinical Correlation

Classical galactosemia

Enzyme deficiency: Galactose-1-phosphate uridyltransferase is deficient in classical galactosemia.

Clinical presentation: Bilateral cataract, mental retardation (due to repeated hypoglycemia), liver enlargement (hepatomegaly).

Benign galactosemia

Enzyme deficiency: Galactokinase is deficient in benign galactosemia.

Clinical presentation: Bilateral cataract.

Key Notes

6

Fructose Metabolism

Key concepts

- Fructose is metabolized in liver as well as extrahepatic tissues.
- Pathway in liver requires **fructokinase** enzyme which converts fructose to fructose-1-phosphate, and in extrahepatic cell **hexokinase** converts fructose to fructose-6-phosphate.
- Ultimate fate of fructose during its metabolism is glycolytic steps where pyruvate is produced.

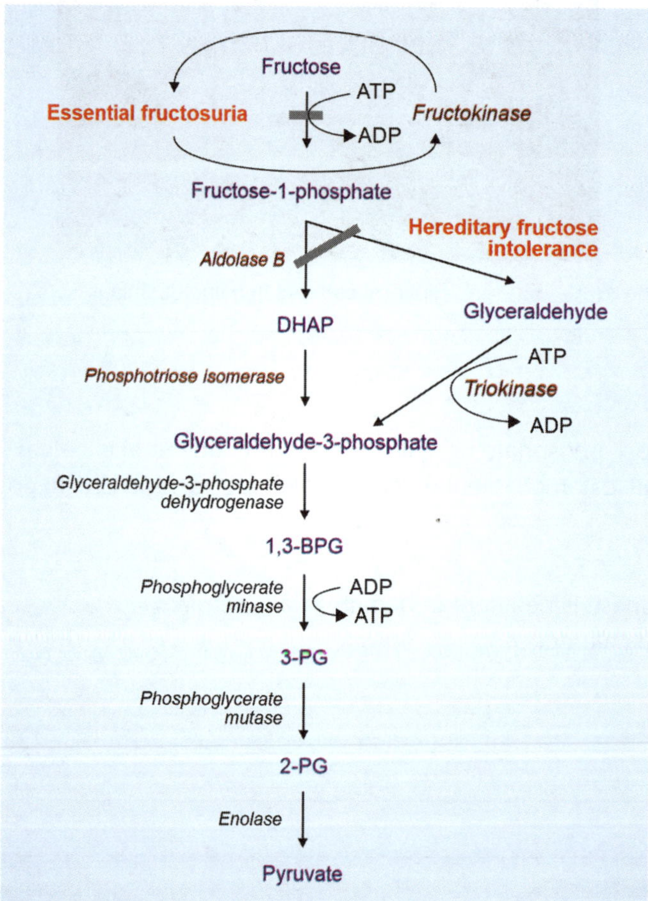

Fig. 6.1: Fructose metabolism in liver

Enzyme Defect in Fructose Catabolism

- *Hereditary fructose intolerance:* Enzyme defect is aldolase B.
- *Benign fructosuria:* Enzyme defect is fructokinase.

Key Notes

7

HMP Shunt Pathway

HEXOSE MONOPHOSPHATE SHUNT

Also known as pentose phosphate pathway (PPP)/Dickens-Horecker pathway/phosphogluconate oxidative pathway.

Key concepts for HMP shunt pathway

- HMP shunt pathway is the cytosolic pathway for glucose oxidation
- Significance of HMP shunt pathway
  - HMP shunt pathway is utilized for production of NADPH and ribose-5 phosphate.
  - NADPH is utilized for reductive biosynthesis and is important to tackle free radicals.
  - Ribose-5-phosphate is needed for synthesis of purine and pyrimidine nucleotide.

Location: Erythrocytes, liver, lactating mammary gland, adipose tissue, adrenal cortex (cytosol).

Clinical Correlation of HMP Shunt Pathway

- Deficiency of G6PD enzyme results in hemolytic anemia due to free radical damage of RBC membrane.

Key Notes

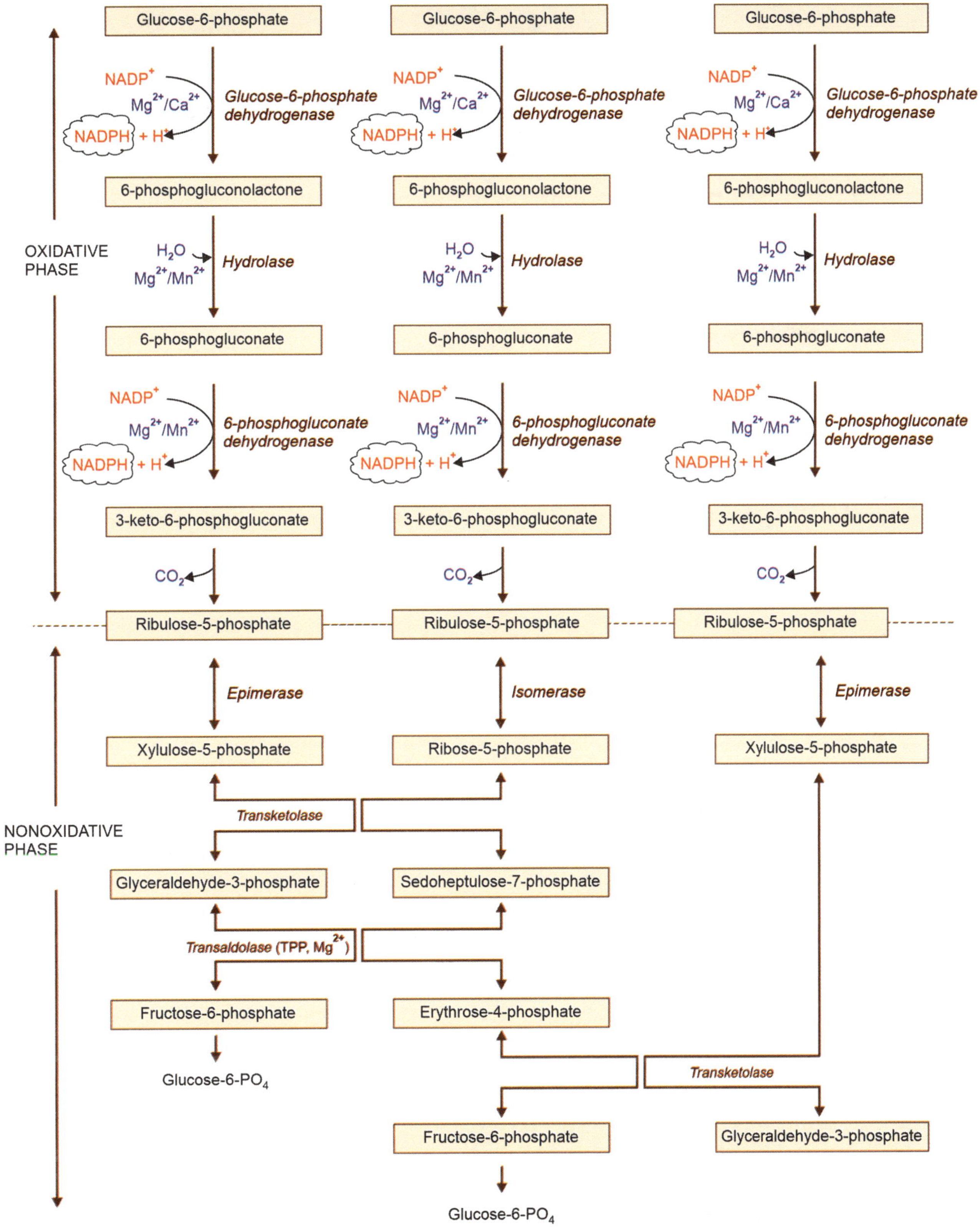

Fig. 7.1: Steps of HMP pathway

8

Uronic Acid Pathway

Key concepts

- Uronic acid pathway occurs in liver.
- Here glucose is oxidized for production of glucuronic acid which is a conjugating agent.
- Unlike lower primates, human is incapable of producing ascorbic acid in uronic acid pathway.
- This is due to absence of L-gulonolactone oxidase enzyme.

Clinical Correlation

- Essential pentosuria is due to deficiency of enzyme xylitol dehydrogenase, which results in excretion of L-xylulose in the urine.

Key Notes

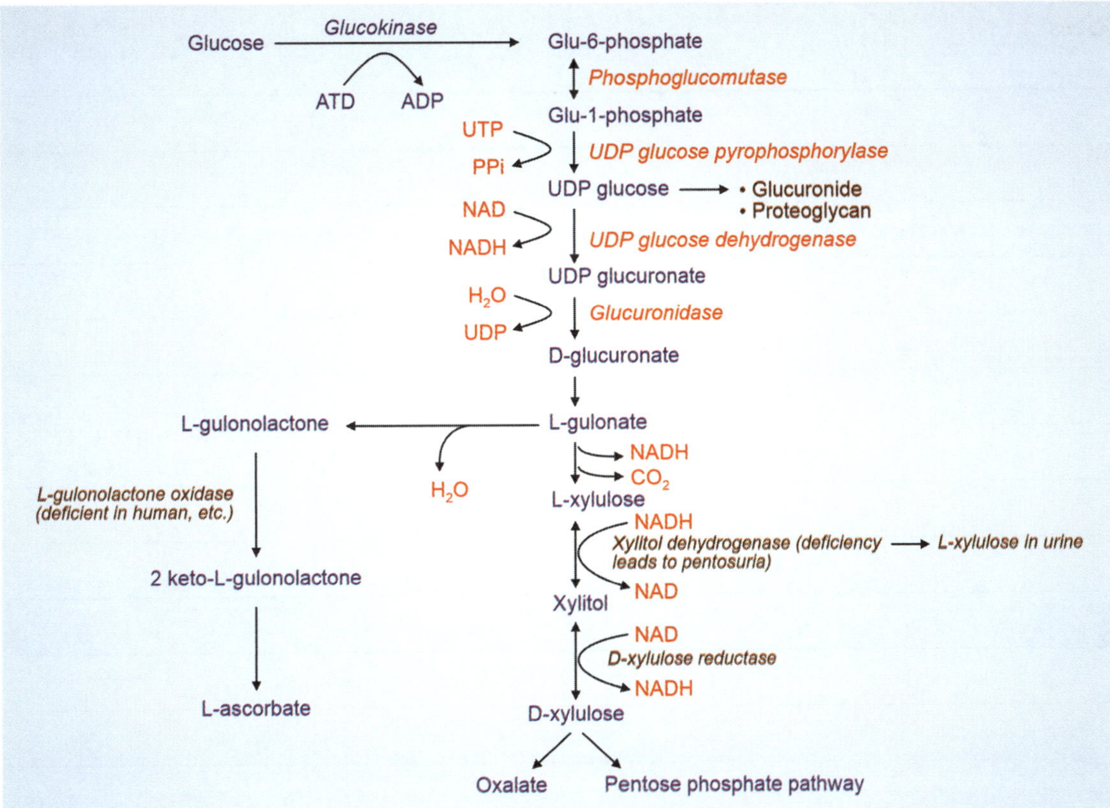

Fig. 8.1: Uronic acid pathway

Key Notes

Key Notes

Key Notes

9 Fatty Acid Synthesis

Key concepts
- Main organ where synthesis of fatty acid takes place is liver.
- *Site:* cytosol

Precursor molecule: It is acetyl-CoA which is generated from glucose and fructose oxidation in well fed state
- Hormone required for synthesis of fatty acid is 'Insulin'.
- Synthesis of fatty acid is the cyclical process where set of four 'reactions' are repeated 'seven' times at the active site of fatty acid synthase complex to generate 16 carbon fatty acid chain (palmitic acid).

The whole process of fatty acid synthesis can be learned under the following headings:
1. Acetyl-CoA and its transportation out of mitochondria.
2. Conversion of acetyl-CoA to malonyl-CoA.
3. Synthesis of fatty acid chain in cyclical reaction.

1. Acetyl-CoA and its Transportation Out of Mitochondria

The condensation of acetyl-CoA to oxaloacetate in the first reaction of the TCA cycle is catalyzed by citrate synthase.

$$\text{Acetyl-CoA} + \text{Oxaloacetate} \rightarrow \text{Citrate}$$

The citrate, thus formed, enters the cytosol with the help of the citrate transporter present on the inner mitochondrial membrane.

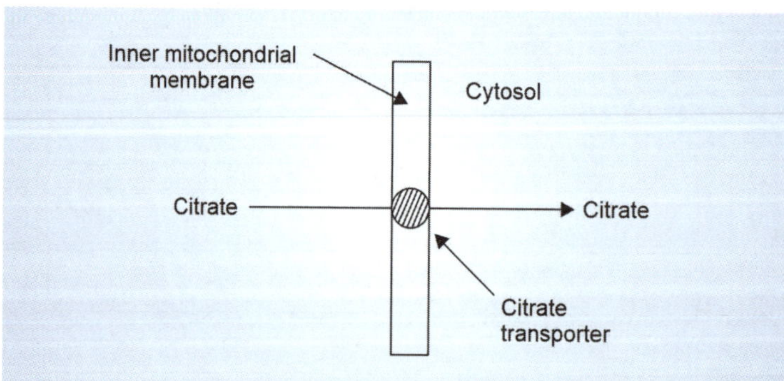

Fig. 9.1: Citrate transporter on IMM

In the cytosol, ' 'the enzyme' ATP citrate lyase' acts upon citrate, which converts citrate into acetyl-CoA and oxaloacetate.

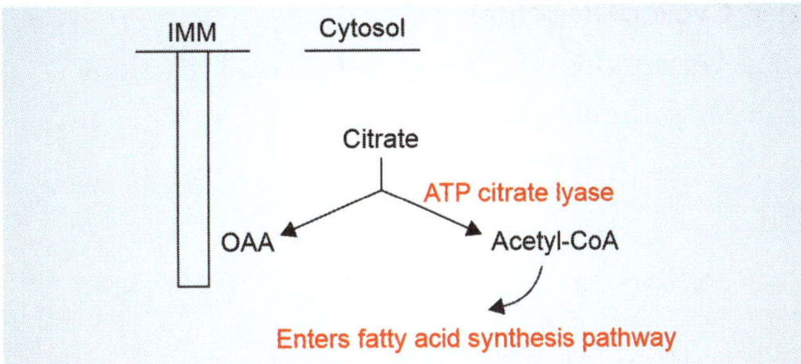

Fig. 9.2: Action of ATP citrate lyase

2. Conversion of Acetyl-CoA to Malonyl-CoA

Acetyl-CoA is the precursor molecule **'the'**, first converted to malonyl-CoA in the cytosol by the 'acetyl-CoA carboxylase' enzyme, the **'rate-limiting 'enzyme'** for fatty acid synthesis.

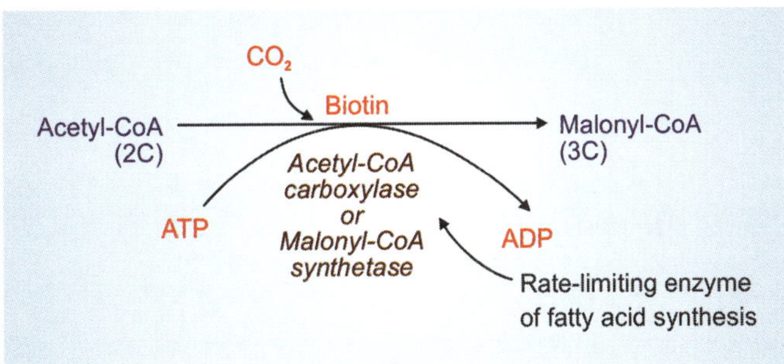

Fig. 9.3: Acetyl-CoA carboxylase activity

FATTY ACID SYNTHASE COMPLEX

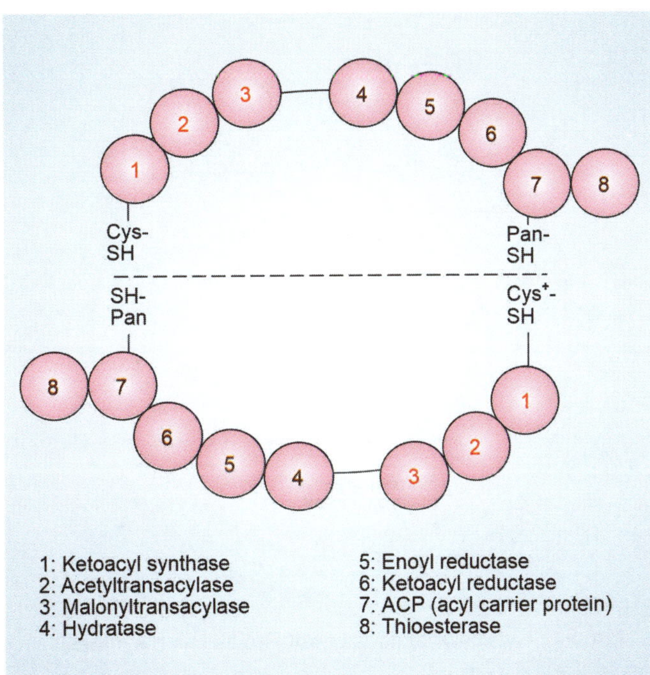

Fig. 9.4: Fatty acid synthase complex

3. Synthesis of Fatty Acid Chain in Cyclical Reaction

Synthesis of palmitic acid (16C) in vertebrates requires seven cyclical reactions.

Each cyclical reaction consists of the following four reactions:

1. Condensation
2. Reduction of carboxyl group
3. Dehydration
4. Reduction of double bond

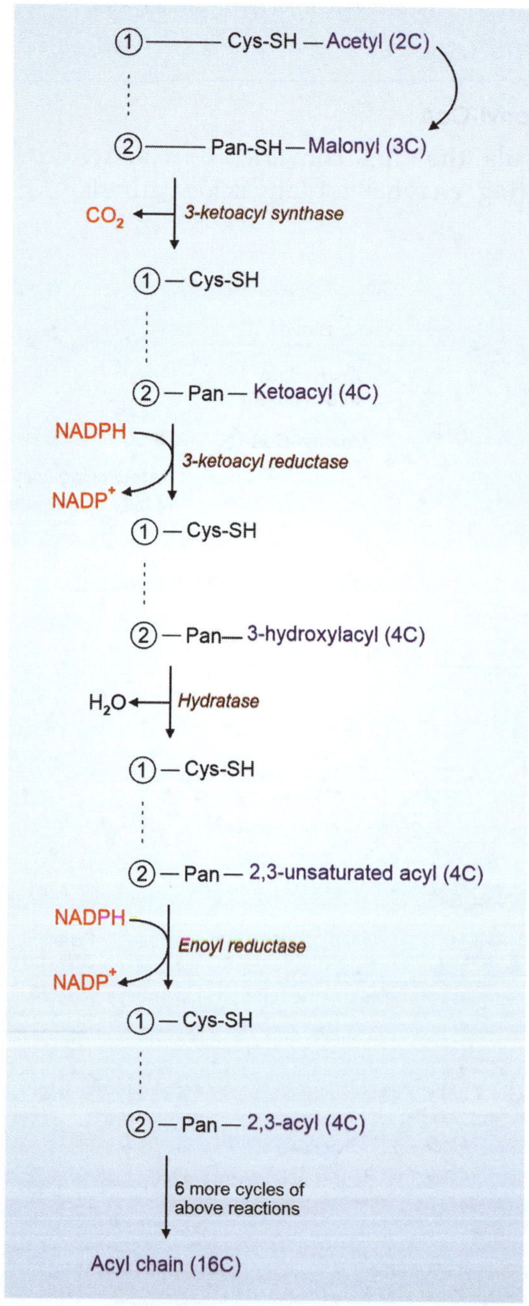

Fig. 9.5: Cyclical reactions of fatty acids chain synthesis

Clinical Correlation

Excess carbohydrate intake results in excessive fatty acid synthesis in the liver, from where it is diverted to extrahepatic tissues like heart and skeletal muscle and adipose cells. In heart and skeletal muscle, fatty acids are immediately oxidized for ATP production, while in adipose cells, these fatty acids where they are stored causing obesity in chronic excessive intake of carbohydrate.

Key Notes

10

Fatty Acid Oxidation

BETA-OXIDATION OF FATTY ACID

> ***Key concepts***
> Beta-oxidation of fatty acid can be discussed under following headings:
> A. *Fatty acid activation (priming of fatty acid) in the cytosol.*
> B. *Transport of fatty acid across the mitochondrial membrane using 'carnitine shuttle'.*
> C. *Cyclical reaction of β-oxidation in the mitochondrial matrix.*

A. Fatty Acid Activation

Acyl-CoA synthetase (or thiokinase) is the enzyme found in the outer mitochondrial membrane. It is the enzyme which is responsible for the activation process of fatty acid via converting it to acyl-CoA.

B. Transport Across the Mitochondrial Membrane/Carnitine Shuttle

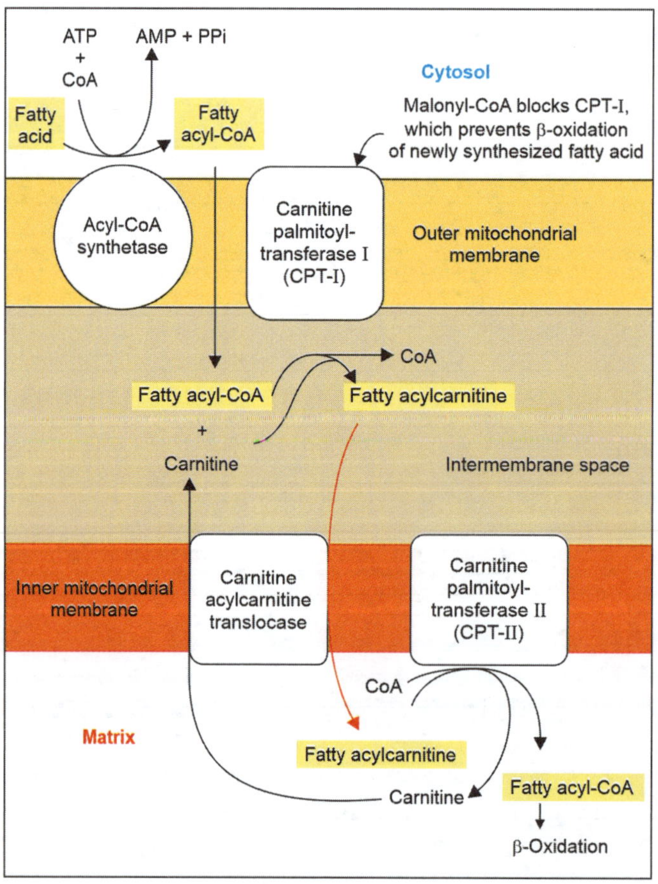

Fig. 10.1: Carnitine shuttle

Clinical Correlation

Deficiency of carnitine seen in

- Preterm babies
- Dialysis
- Liver cirrhosis

Carnitine deficiency results in hypoglycemia as gluconeogenesis does not occur due to lack of β-oxidation of fatty acid.

C. Steps of β-Oxidation of Fatty Acid in Mitochondrial Matrix

Beta-oxidation is a cyclical process where sets of four enzymes catalyze each cycle.

1. Acyl-CoA dehydrogenase
2. Enoyl-CoA hydratase
3. L-hydroxyacyl-CoA dehydrogenase
4. Thiolase

Key Notes

Clinical Correlation

- Medium chain acyl-CoA dehydrogenase deficiency results in frequent hypoglycemia.
- Jamaican vomiting sickness is due to consumption of raw fruit of Akee tree which contains toxin hypoglycin.
- Hybuglycin inhibits medium chain acyl-CoA dehydrogenase resulting in attack of hypoglycin.

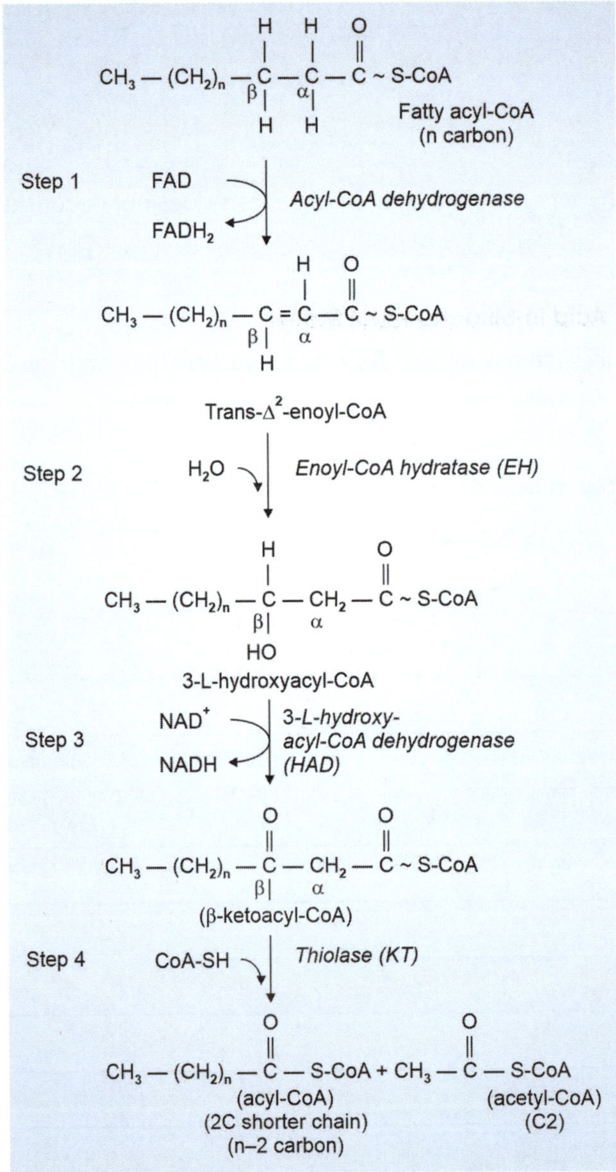

Fig. 10.2: Steps of β-oxidation of fatty acid

Key Notes

d. Alpha-oxidation

This type of oxidation in fatty acid is meant to clear the branch point of branched-chain fatty acids like phytanic acid.

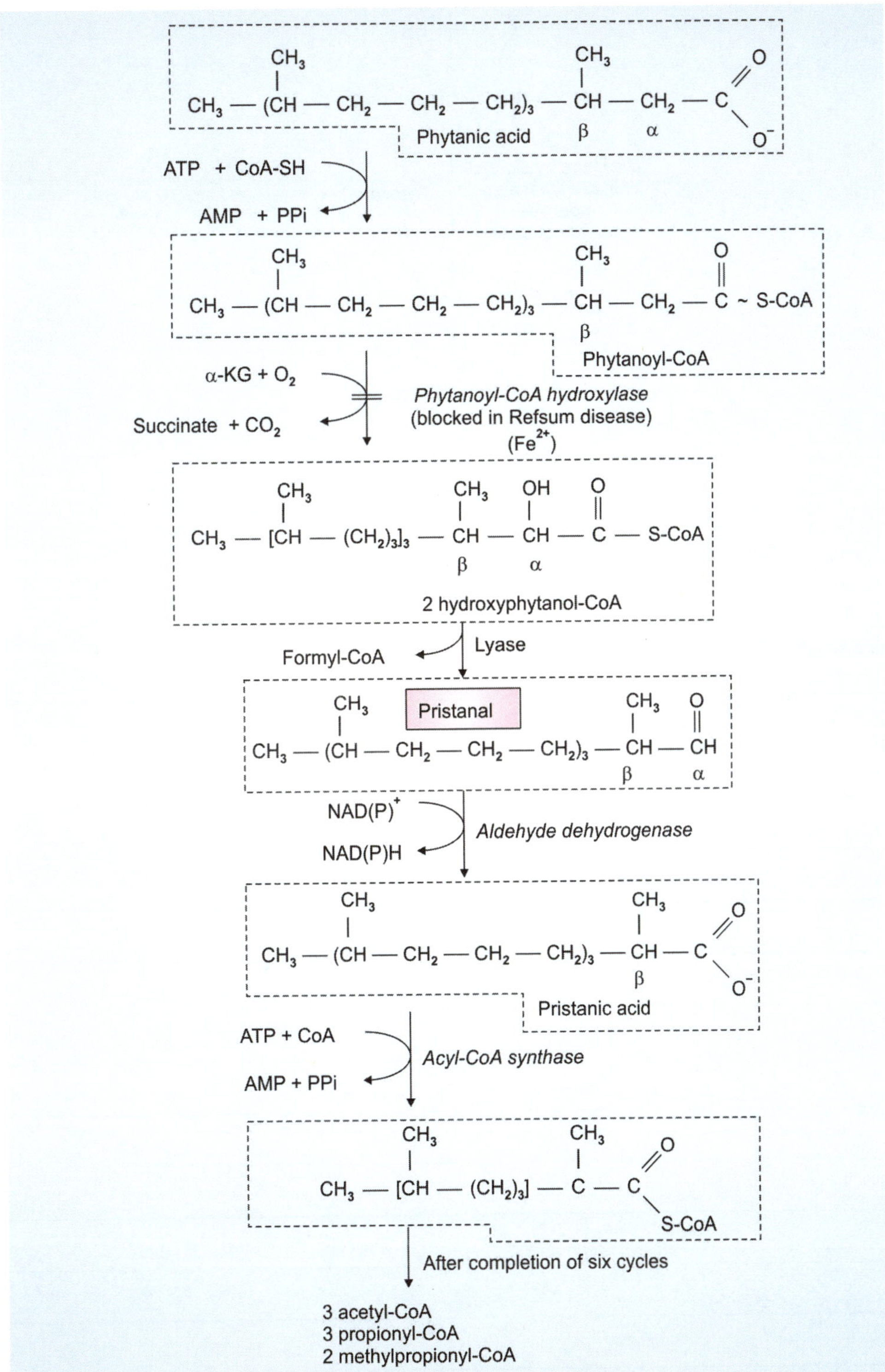

Fig. 10.3: Oxidation of phytanic acid

D. Omega-oxidation

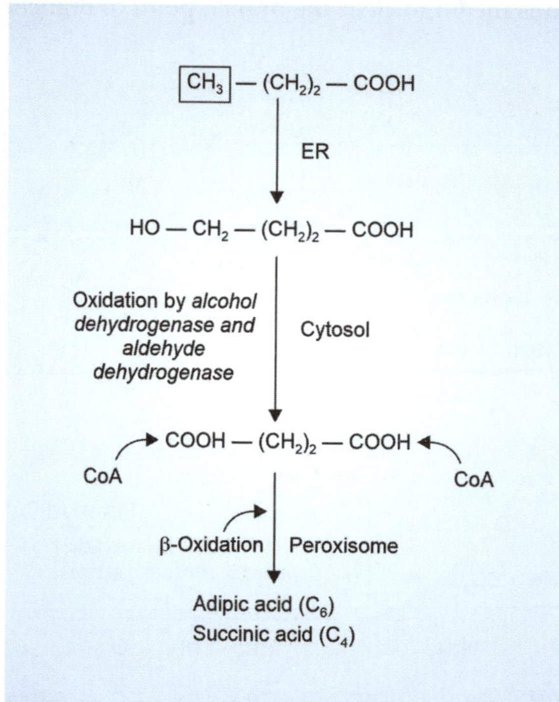

Fig. 10.4: ω-Oxidation pathway

Key Notes

11

Ketone Body Metabolism

Beta-oxidation of fatty acid produces acetyl-CoA, the majority of which is utilized in the TCA cycle for the production of ATP.

Following are the steps involved in the production of ketone body from acetyl-CoA

1. Condensation of two molecules of acetyl-CoA by thiolase enzyme (acetyl-CoA—acetyltransferase enzyme) to produce acetoacetyl-CoA.
2. Condensation of another molecule of acetyl-CoA to acetoacetyl-CoA to produce HMG-CoA by HMG-CoA synthase enzyme.
3. HMG-CoA is degraded to acetoacetate and acetyl-CoA by HMG-CoA lyase enzyme. Acetoacetate is the common precursor of β-hydroxybutyrate and acetone.

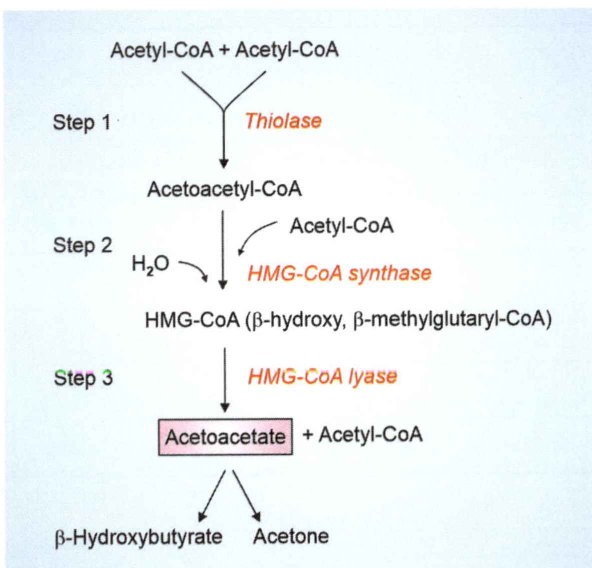

Fig. 11.1: Production of ketone body

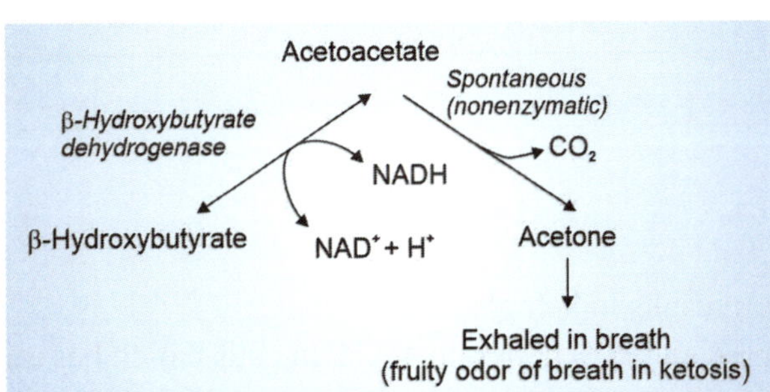

Fig. 11.2: Conversion of acetoacetate at β-hydroxybutyrate and acetone

KETONE BODY UTILIZATION

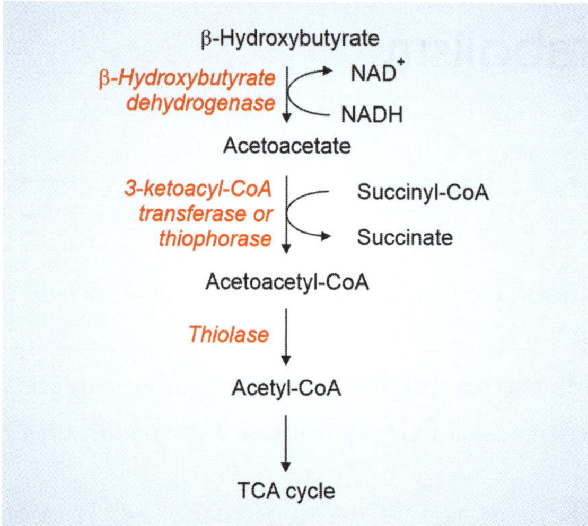

Fig. 11.3: Utilization of acetoacetate and β-hydroxybutyrate at peripheral tissues

Key Notes

Clinical Correlation

- Excessive fatty acid β-oxidation results in ketogenesis.
- Ketone body is the fuel which is capable of generating ATP in cells which has mitochondria and all the enzymes required for ketolysis.
- Excess concentration of ketone body in blood results in ketoacidosis.

12

Cholesterol and Bile Acid Synthesis

Cholesterol is 27-carbon compound with a ring structure.

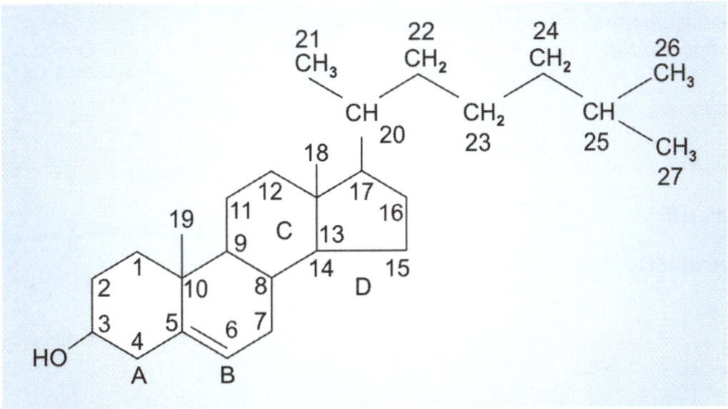

Fig. 12.1: Structure of cholesterol: 27-carbon compound

Key Notes

The whole process of cholesterol biogenesis is divided into four stages

a. Acetyl-CoA producing 6-carbon compound mevalonate.
b. Conversion of 6-carbon mevalonate to 5-carbon isoprenoid units.
c. Condensation of six isoprenoids to form 30-carbon squalene.
d. Conversion of squalene to cholesterol.

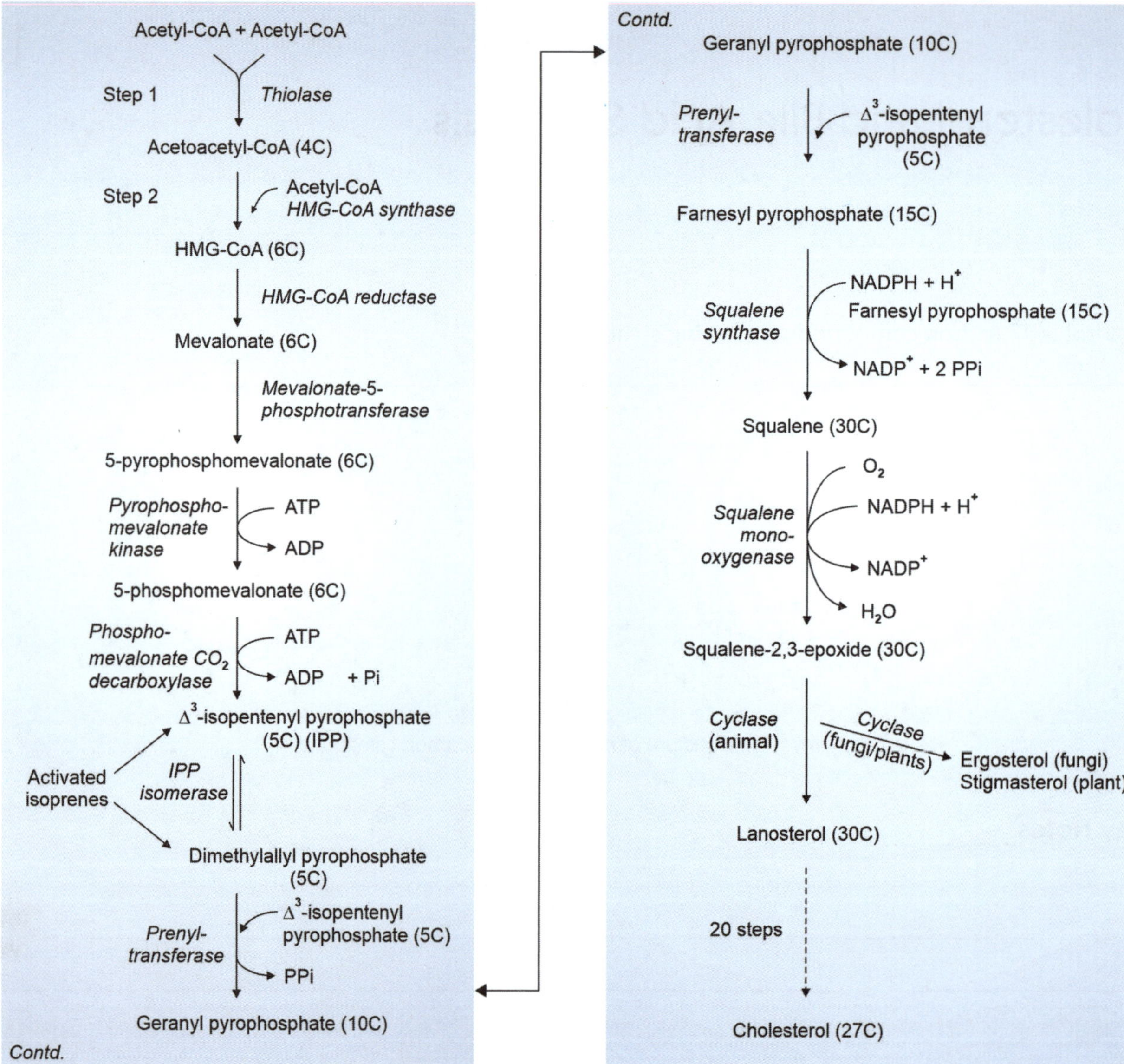

Fig. 12.2: Steps of biosynthesis of cholesterol

Key Notes

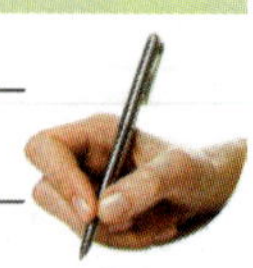

Conversion of Cholesterol to Bile Acid

Excess cholesterol is converted to bile acid and excreted. Bile acids are broadly of two types.

1. Primary bile acids
2. Secondary bile acids

7α-hydroxylation of cholesterol is the first committed step in the biosynthesis of bile acid, and it also acts as a rate-limiting step for the synthesis of bile acid.

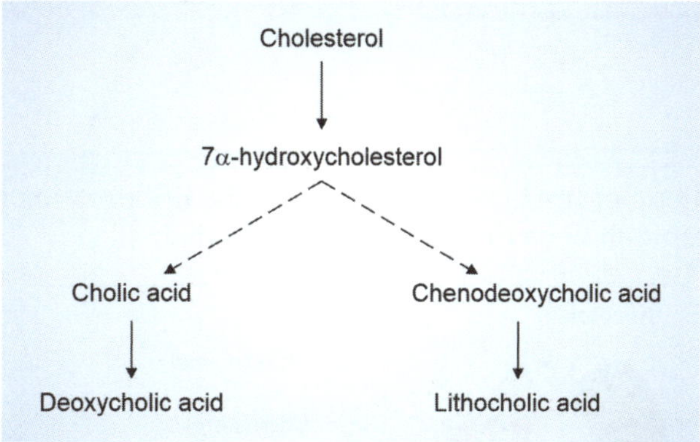

Fig. 12.3: Primary and secondary bile acids

Key Notes

13

Lipoprotein Metabolism (Chylomicron, VLDL, LDL and HDL Metabolism)

LIPOPROTEIN METABOLISM

Lipoproteins are structures made up of lipids and proteins. All the lipoproteins possess an inner core filled with nonpolar lipids and an amphipathic shell having amphipathic lipids in it.

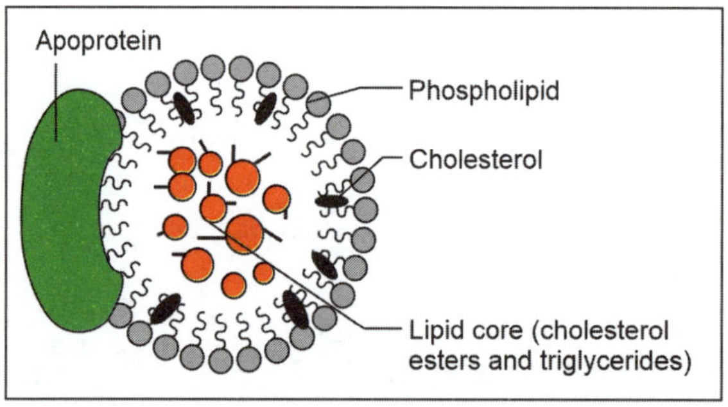

Fig. 13.1: Structure of a typical lipoprotein

Key concept in chylomicron and VLDL metabolism

- Chylomicrons (CMs) are organized in intestinal mucosa. Formation of chylomicron is an attempt to absorb dietary lipids to the blood circulation.
- Chylomicrons carry exogenous/dietary lipids to peripheral tissues.
- VLDL is synthesized in liver and is metabolized in blood circulation in a pattern similar to chylomicron metabolism.
- Lipoprotein lipase enzyme which is adherent to capillary endothelial wall is the key enzyme for metabolism of chylomicron and VLDL metabolism.
- Lipoprotein lipase is activated by ApoC-I and ApoC-II.
- Lipoprotein lipase acts on core triacylglycerol and release its fatty acid which is supplied to tissues.
- CM remnant is cleared from plasma and VLDL remnant (IDL) is either directly cleared from circulation or is converted to LDL and is further metabolized.

Key Notes

CHYLOMICRON METABOLISM

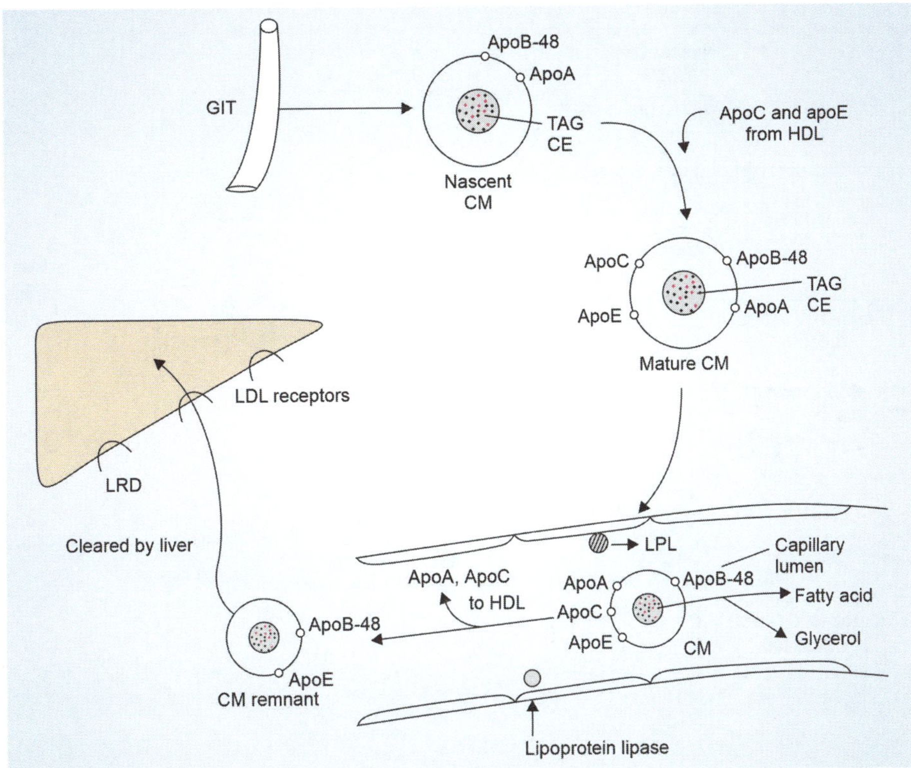

Fig. 13.2: Chylomicron metabolism

Key Notes

VLDL METABOLISM

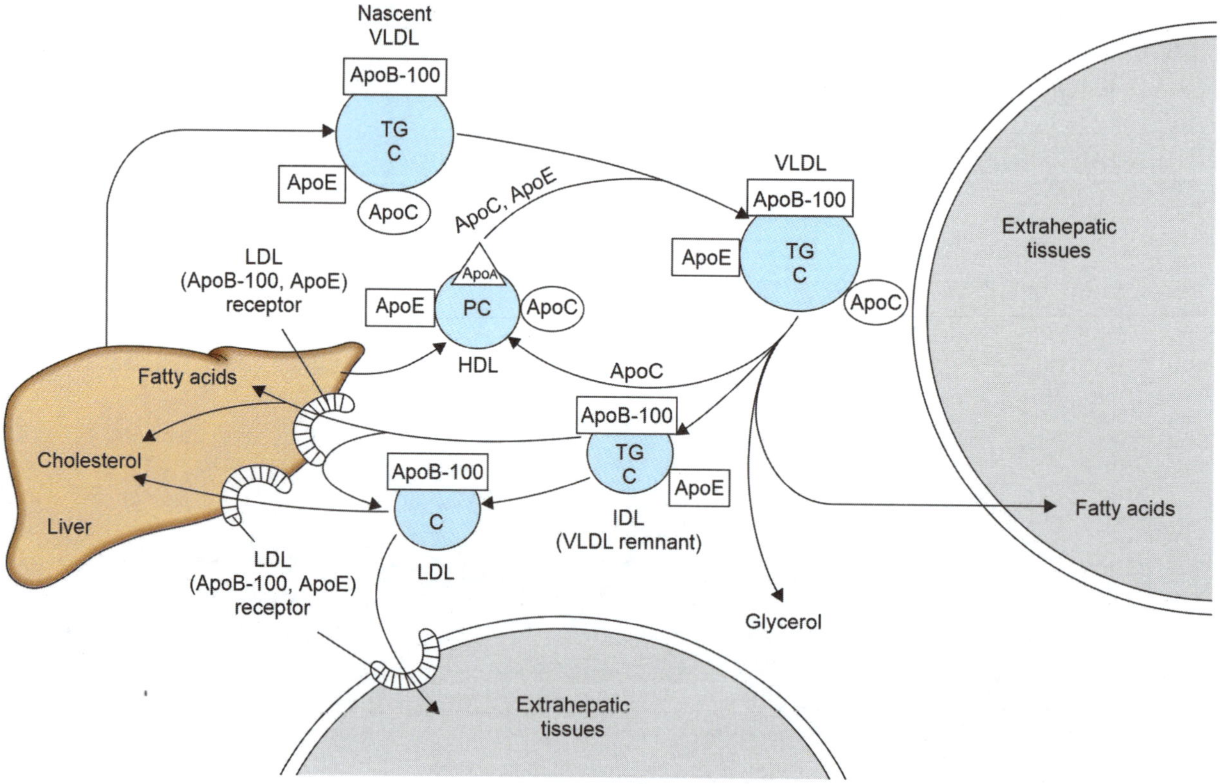

Fig. 13.3: Outline of VLDL metabolism

Clinical Correlation/Chylomicron and VLDL

- Deficiency of lipoprotein lipase or its activator ApoC results in hyper-tri-acyl-glyceredemia
- Type I hyper-tri-acyl-glyceredemia deficiency of lipoprotein lipase enzyme
- Type V
- Deficiency of ApoC

Key Notes

LDL METABOLISM

Key concepts/LDL metabolism

- LDL is synthesized from VLDL during its metabolism.
- LDL is responsible for delivering cholesterol to extrahepatic tissues.
- LDL receptors identify ApoB-100 protein present on LDL particle and endocytose LDL.

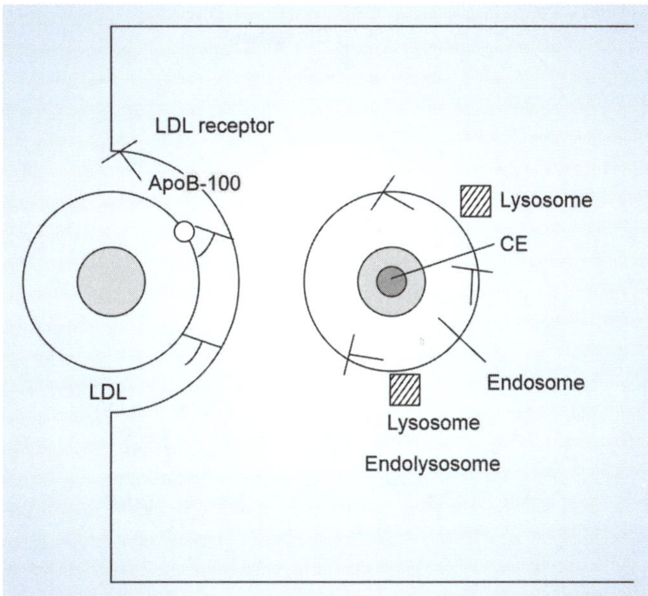

Fig. 13.4: Recognition of LDL by LDL receptors at extrahepatic tissues

Clinical Correlation/LDL Metabolism

- Defective clearance of LDL from the plasma results in accumulation of LDL in the plasma (either due to mutation of LDL receptor or mutated ApoB-100) which is reflected as hypercholesterolemia in lipid profile.

Key Notes

HDL METABOLISM

Key concept of HDL metabolism

- Liver and intestine synthesize and secrete disk-shaped nascent HDL particle, which is known as discoidal HDL.
- Discoidal HDL is a flattened structure having shell of phospholipid and free cholesterol.
- Most abundant type of phospholipid in the shell of HDL is lecithin.

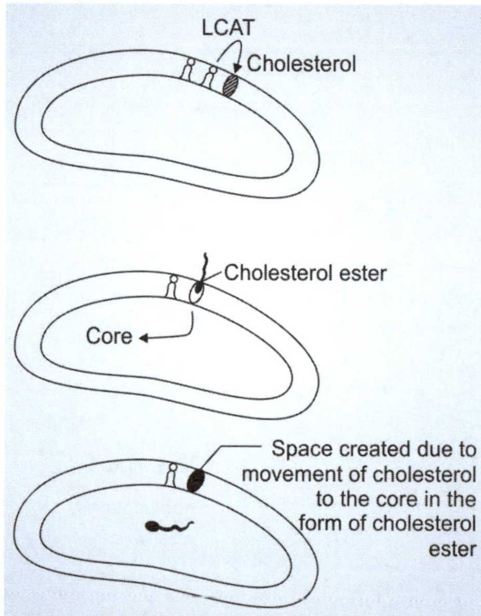

Fig. 13.5: Action of LCAT on HDL shell

Key Notes

DYSLIPIDEMIA

Table 13.1: Fredrickson classification of hyperlipoproteinemia

Type	Metabolic defect	Elevated lipoprotein	TAG level	Cholesterol level	Inheritance
Type I (Familial hyper-tri-acyl-glyceredemia)	Lipoprotein lipase	↑CM	↑↑	Ⓝ	AR
Type IIa (Familial hypercholes-terolemia)	LDL receptor mutation or ApoB gene mutation	↑LDL	Ⓝ	↑↑	AD
Type IIb	Defect as in IIa, additionally increased VLDL secretion	↑LDL ↑VLDL	↑	↑↑	AD
Type III (remnant removal disease)	Abnormal ApoE (E_2)	• Increased CM remnant • Increased VLDL remnant (IDL)	↑	↑↑	AR
Type IV (Familial-combined hyperlipidemia)	Overproduction of VLDL	↑VLDL	↑↑	↑	Polygenic combined hyperlipidemia
Type V	Deficiency of ApoC-II	↑VLDL ↑CM	↑↑	N	AR

Key Notes

Section C

Amino Acids and their Metabolism

14

Urea Cycle (Krebs-Henseleit Cycle or Ornithine Cycle)

The urea cycle is responsible for urea production from amino groups of amino acids.

The amino group of amino acids reaches the liver via glutamate. Glutamate accumulates the amino group from amino acid via transamination reaction and delivers it to the liver via deamination.

Transamination

The transfer of an amino group from an amino acid to a keto acid is known as transamination. Transamination is catalyzed by the transaminase enzyme.

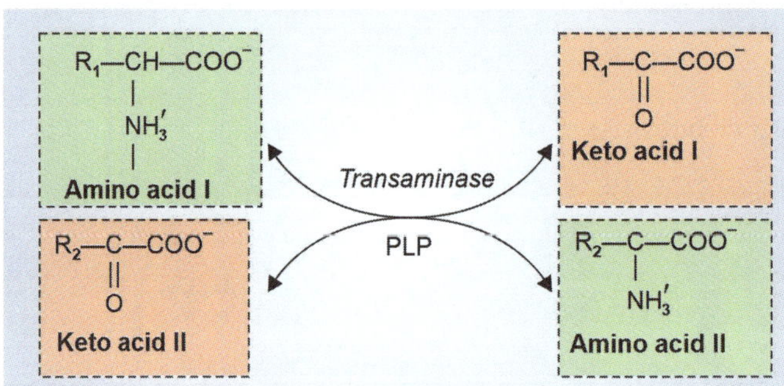

Fig. 14.1: Transamination

Deamination

Removing amino groups from the amino acid as ammonia is called deamination. The liberation of free ammonia from the amino group of amino acids when coupled with oxidation is known as oxidative deamination.

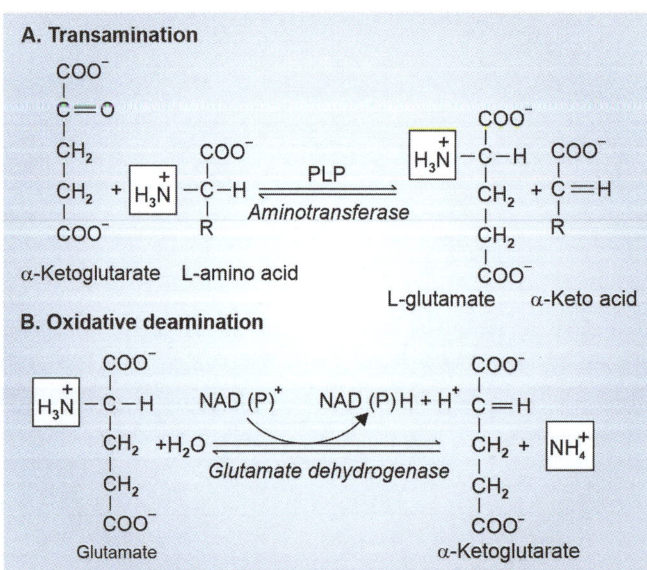

Fig. 14.2: Transamination and oxidative deamination

Urea Cycle Reactions

Reactions of the urea cycle are partly mitochondrial and cytosolic.

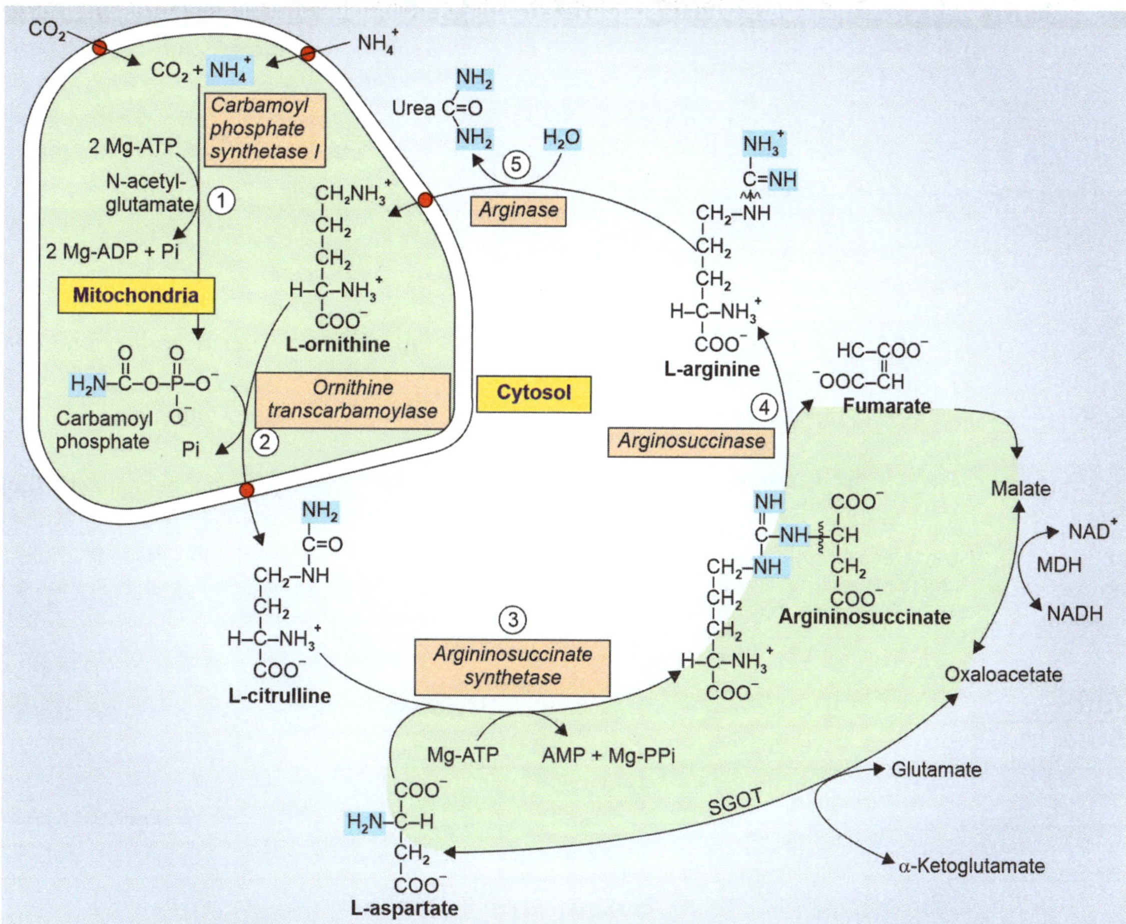

Fig. 14.3: Urea cycle

Key Notes

Disorders of the Urea Cycle

Mutation in any of the enzymes in the urea cycle results in urea cycle disorder characterized by hyperammonemia and its associated manifestation. They are summarised below.

Table 14.1: Urea cycle disorders with respective enzyme deficiencies and clinical presentation

S. No.	Urea cycle enzyme defect	Condition	Inheri-tance	Clinical features
1.	Carbamoyl phosphate synthase 1	Carbamoyl phosphate synthase 1 deficiency (hyperammonemia type I)	AR	Lethargy, coma, aversion to protein, intellectual disability, hyperammonemia
2.	N-acetylglutamate synthase	N-acetylglutamate synthase deficiency	AR	-do-
3.	Ornithine transcarbamoylase (OTC)	OTC deficiency (hyperammonemia type II)	XL	-do-
4.	Argininosuccinate synthase	Citrullinemia type 1	AR	-do-
5.	Argininosuccinate lyase	Argininosuccinic acidemia or argininosuccinate urea	AR	-do- and trichorrhexis nodosa
6.	Arginase	Arginase deficiency	AR	Spastic tetraparesis, microcephaly, mental retardation
7.	Mitochondrial ornithine carrier—ORNT1	HHH syndrome	AR	Hyperammonemia, hyperornithinemia, homocitrullinemia
8.	Mitochondrial aspartate/ glutamate carrier—CTLN2 (citrin deficiency)	Citrullinemia type 2	AR	Neonatal intrahepatic cholestasis, behavioral change, stupor, coma

Key Notes

Simple, Hydroxyl and Branched-chain Amino Acid (Glycine, Alanine, Serine, Threonine, Leucine, Valine and Isoleucine)

15

GLYCINE

A. Synthesis of Glycine

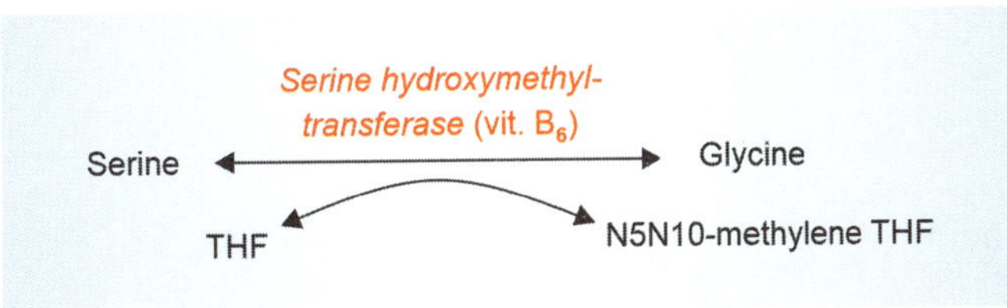

Fig. 15.1: Glycine synthesis from serine

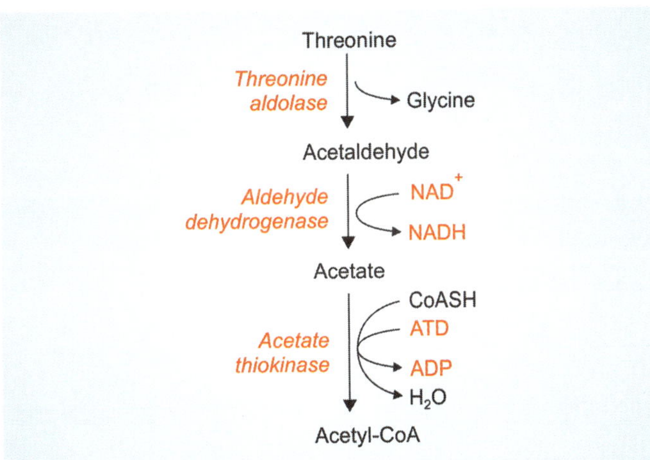

Fig. 15.2: Threonine aldolase

B. Uses of Glycine

Glycine is Utilized in the Following Aspects

a. Purine *de novo* biosynthesis (C4, C5, N7 atoms of purine ring are donated from glycine)
b. Glutathione synthesis (γ-glutamyl-cysteinyl-glycine) needs glutamic acid, cysteine and glycine.
c. Heme biosynthesis (glycine and succinyl-CoA are precursors)
d. Creatine (glycine + arginine + methionine)
e. Glycine as a neurotransmitter
f. Conjugation with bile acids (glycocholic acid and glycochenodeoxycholic acid), which increases amphipathic properties of bile acid.
g. Detoxification of benzoic acid by synthesis of hippuric acid.
h. Collagen formation (every third residue in collagen polypeptide is glycine)

ALANINE

a. A nonessential glucogenic amino acid.
b. Alanine is quantitatively the most important amino acid taken up by the liver from peripheral tissues, especially from skeletal muscles, during protein degradation.

SERINE

Serine is a nonessential glucogenic amino acid.

It is synthesized from:

a. 3-phosphoglycerate (an intermediate of the glycolysis)
b. Glycine: Via serine hydroxymethyltransferase enzyme.

Serine Contributes to the Formation of the Following Compounds

- Glycine
- Cysteine
- Alanine
- Phosphatidylserine
- Selenocysteine (21st amino acid)

Selenocysteine is Found at the Active Site of the Following Enzymes

- Thioredoxin reductase
- Glutathione peroxidase
- Deiodinase
- Glycine reductase
- Selenoprotein P

Key Notes

BRANCHED-CHAIN AMINO ACID CATABOLISM

There are three amino acids that have branching in their side chain. They are:

- Valine
- Leucine
- Isoleucine

During the degradation of the branched-chain amino acid, the first three metabolic reactions are common to all three amino acids. These three reactions are:

1. Transamination
2. Oxidative decarboxylation
3. FAD-dependent dehydrogenation

Key Notes

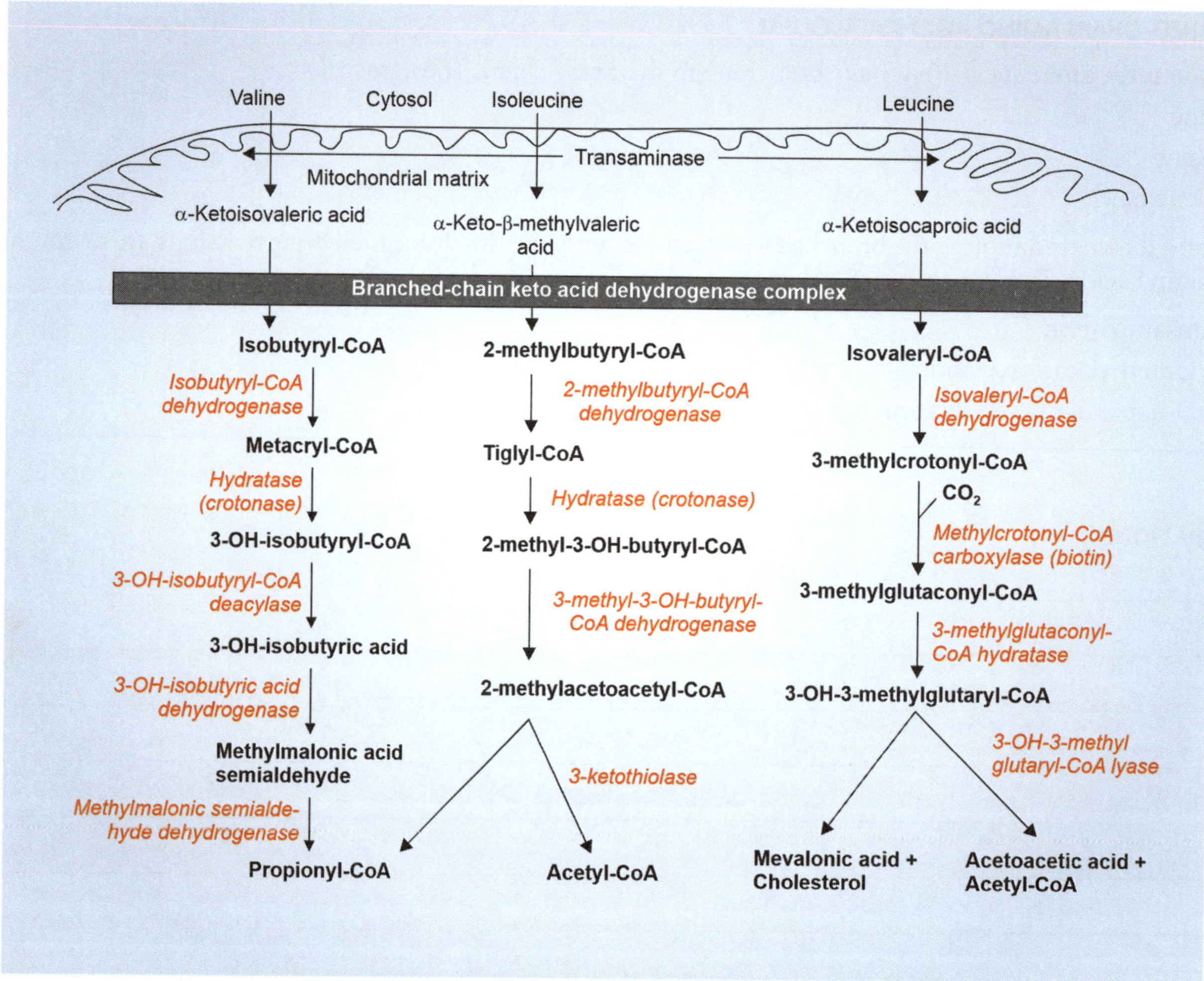

Fig. 15.3: Branched-chain amino acid metabolism

Metabolic Defects in Branched-chain Amino Acid Degradation

a. Maple syrup urine disease (MSUD) (also known as branched-chain ketonuria): Due to defect of branched-chain α-keto acid dehydrogenase complex.
b. Intermittent branched-chain ketonuria.
c. Isovaleric aciduria: Due to defect of isovaleryl-CoA dehydrogenase enzyme.

Key Notes

16 Acidic and Basic Amino Acids (Aspartic Acid, Glutamic Acid, Arginine, Lysine and Histidine)

ACIDIC AMINO ACIDS

GLUTAMIC ACID

Importance of Glutamic Acid

- Glutamic acid is the excitatory neurotransmitter, and its α-decarboxylation gives rise to γ-aminobutyric acid (GABA), an inhibitory neurotransmitter.
- Glutamate fixes NH_3 in the brain and intestine with the help of glutamine synthetase enzyme.
- Glutaminase enzyme found in renal tubular cells releases NH_3 from glutamine, which helps in maintaining acid–base balance via accepting H^+ from the urine and forming NH_4^+.
- Glutamine provides nitrogen for forming arginine, carbamoyl phosphate and purine nucleotide.

ASPARTIC ACID

Key Notes

BASIC AMINO ACID

Basic amino acids are arginine, lysine and histidine.

ARGININE

Synthesis: Arginine is synthesized from glutamate in the following reaction:

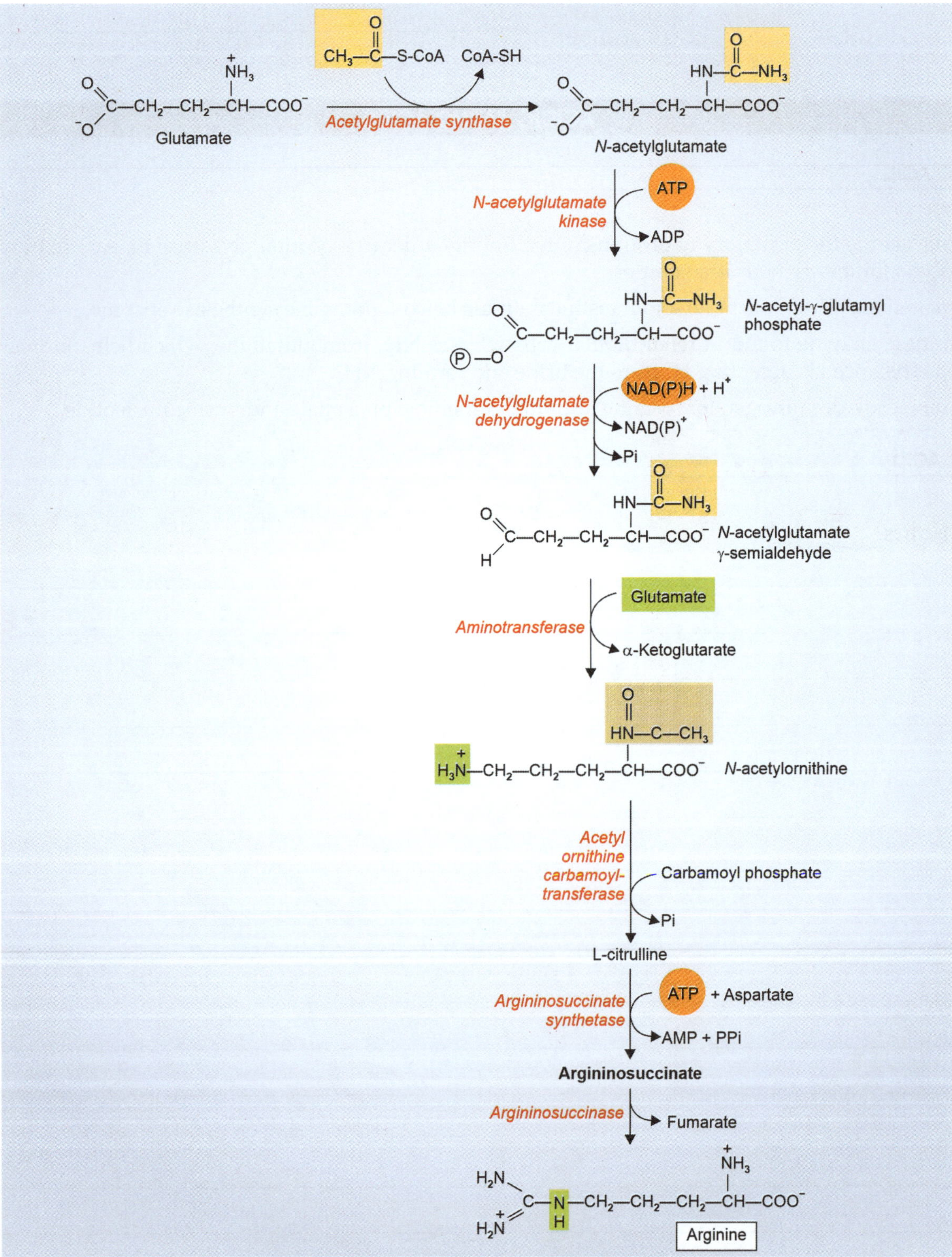

Fig. 16.1: Synthesis of arginine from glutamate

Catabolism

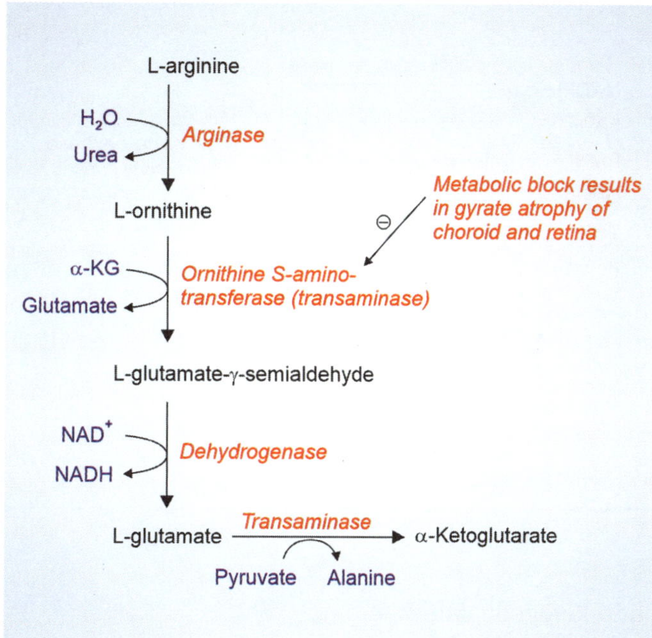

Fig. 16.2: Catabolism of arginine

Special products of arginine

1. Creatine
2. Nitric oxide
3. Urea formation

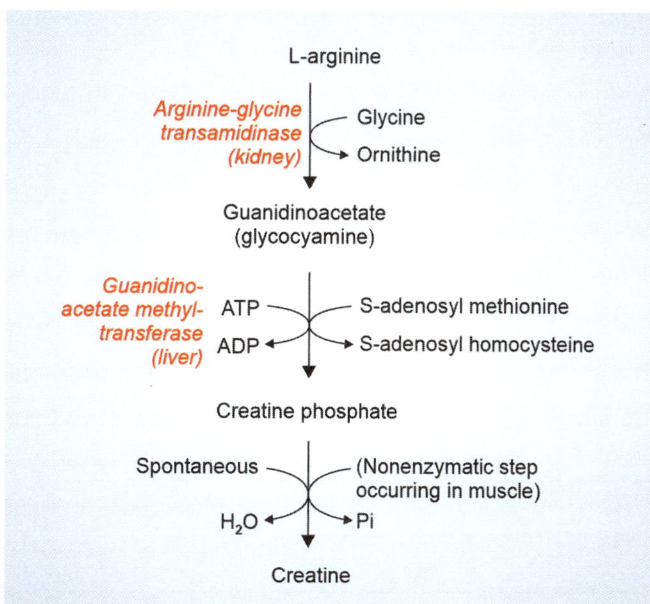

Fig. 16.3: Creatine synthesis from arginine

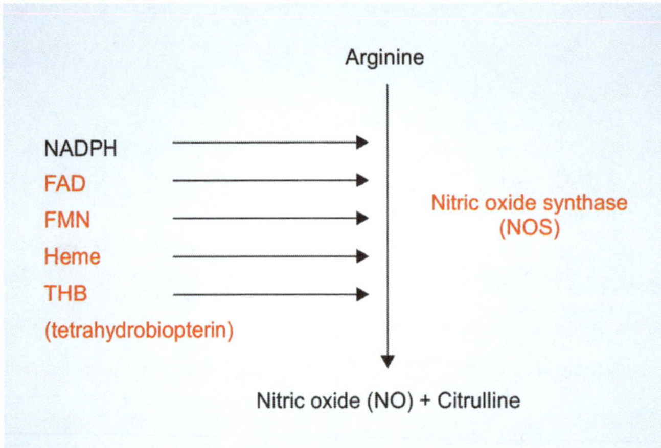

Fig. 16.4: Synthesis of nitric oxide from arginine

LYSINE

1. Lysine is basic amino acid
2. Lysine is essential amino acid
3. Lysine has both glucogenic and ketogenic fate
4. Lysine is required to synthesize carnitine

HISTIDINE

1. Histidine is semi-essential amino acid
2. Histidine is gluconeogenic amino acid.

FIGLU EXCRETION TEST (HISTIDINE LOAD TEST OR HISTIDINE STRESS TEST)

This test is done to find out latent folic acid deficiency.

Excretion of more than 30 mg of FIGLU in 24-hour urine after giving 15 gm of histidine per orally in divided doses indicates latent folic acid deficiency.

Key Notes

17

Sulphur-containing Amino Acid (Methionine, Cysteine and Homocysteine)

METHIONINE METABOLISM

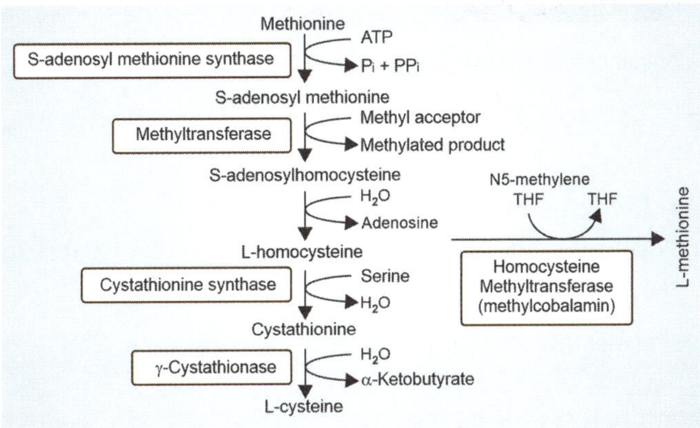

Fig. 17.1: Methionine metabolism and fate of homocysteine

METHIONINE IS AN ESSENTIAL AMINO ACID

Methionine synthesizes cysteine in a multistep process.

SAM (S-adenosyl methionine) is an important intermediate during methionine metabolism which provides methyl group in various metabolic reactions.

Key Notes

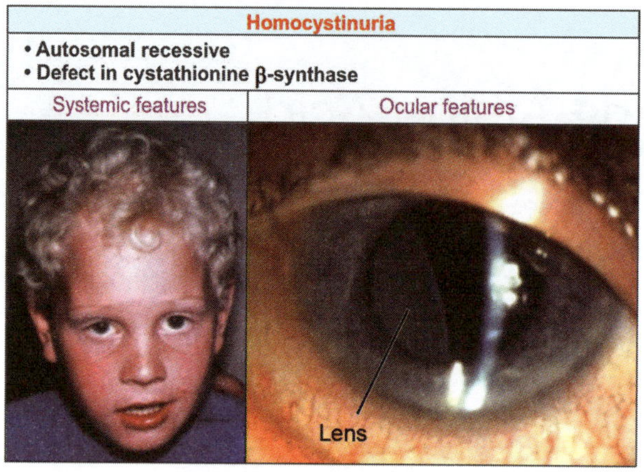

Fig. 17.2: Clinical presentation of HCU. Note: Fine wooly hair and subluxation lens

Homocystinuria is a disease related to defective methionine metabolism where large amount of homocystine is excreted in the urine.

This disease is characterized by involvement of

Ocular system: Subluxation lens, optic atrophy, secondary glaucoma and retinal detachment.

Central nervous system

- Cerebellar ataxia, nystagmus, aphasia, hypotonia and muscle weakness.
- Vascular system
- Atherosclerosis and thromboembolic episode.

Skeletal System

- Arachnodactyly
- Osteoporosis
- Scoliosis

Types of homocystinuria

Type I: Due to deficiency of cystathione β-synthase

Type II: Due to deficiency of cystathionase

Type III: Due to deficiency of N5N10 methylene tetrahydrofolate reductase.

Key Notes

18

One-Carbon Metabolism

ONE-CARBON POOL

Different groups containing one-carbon are collectively known as one-carbon groups.

These are:

1. Formyl group (–CHO)
2. Formimino group (–CH = NH)
3. Methyl group ($-CH_3$)
4. Methylene group ($-CH_2^-$)
5. Methenyl group (= CH–)
6. Hydroxymethyl group ($-CH_2OH$)
7. Carbon dioxide (CO_2)

> ***Key concept***
>
> **Source of one-carbon compound in one-carbon pool**
>
> One-carbon groups or compounds are contributed in one-carbon pool by following amino acids:
>
> 1. Serine (major contributor): N5N10-methylene THFA
> 2. Glycine: N5N10-methylene THFA
> 3. Histidine: N5-formimino THFA
> 4. Tryptophan: N10-formyl THFA
> 5. Choline: N5-hydroxymethyl THFA
> 6. Serine is the major contributor of one-carbon group
>
> **Utilization of one-carbon group**
>
> One-carbon units are used for the synthesis of following compounds:
>
> 1. C2 and C8 of purine
> 2. Synthesis of thymine base
> 3. Formylation of methionyl tRNA
> 4. Synthesis of serine from glycine
> 5. Synthesis of methionine from homocysteine by homocysteine methyltransferase enzyme.
> 6. *Transmethylation reaction:* During synthesis of creatine, choline and epinephrine.

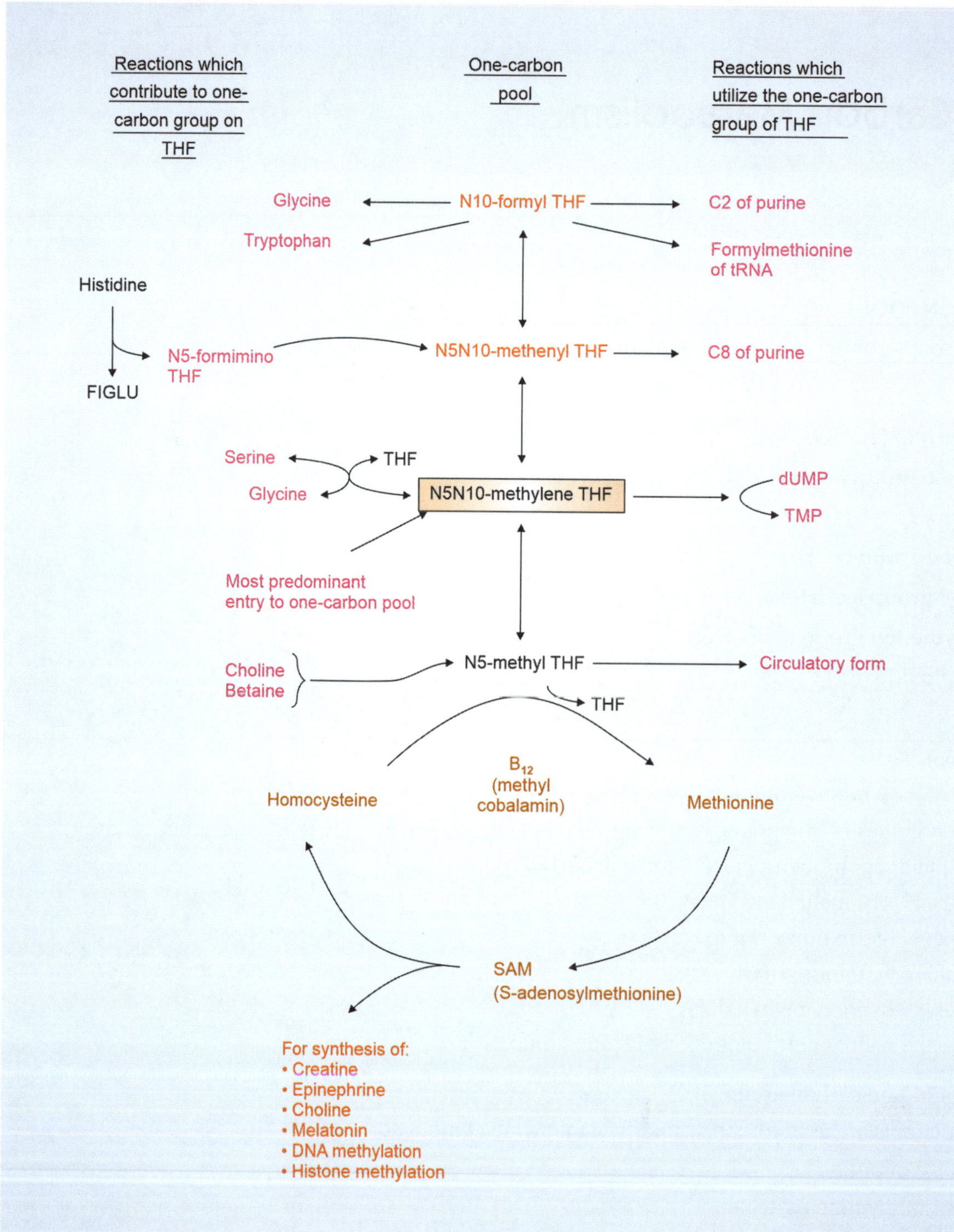

Fig. 18.1: One-carbon metabolism

Key Notes

Aromatic Amino Acid (Phenylalanine, Tyrosine and Tryptophan)

- Phenylalanine, tyrosine and tryptophan are aromatic amino acids.
- All above three amino acids are both glucogenic and ketogenic.

Key concept

Phenylalanine

- Phenylalanine is an essential amino acid. Most of dietary phenylalanine is converted to tyrosine in human system in a biochemical reaction, where hydroxyl group is added the side chain benzene ring of phenylalanine, converting it to phenol.
- Reaction is catalyzed by phenylalanine hydroxylase which uses molecular oxygen and a source of hydrogen, 'tetrahydrobiopterin (THB)'.

Key Notes

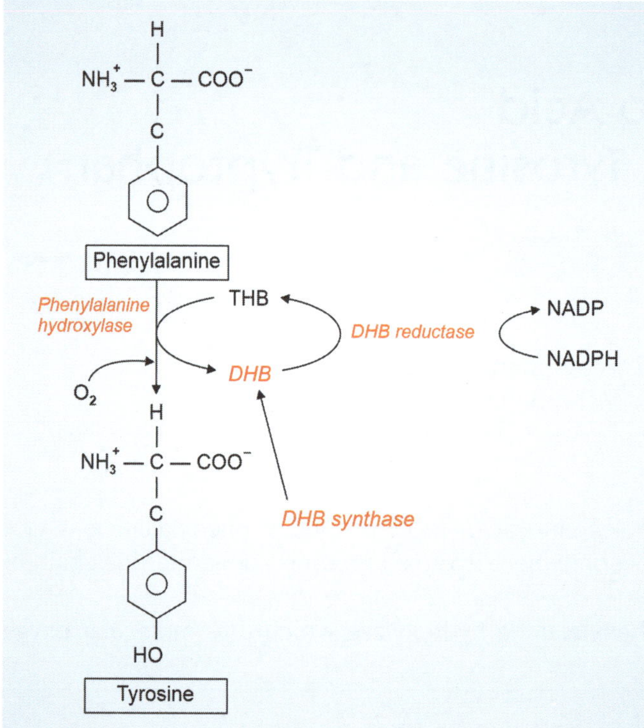

Fig. 19.1: Synthesis of tyrosine from phenylalanine

Phenylketonuria (PKU)

Metabolic defect in conversion of phenylalanine to tyrosine results in phenylketonuria.

Diagnosis of PKU

1. *Blood phenylalanine level:* Level of phenylalanine in blood is increased to >20 mg/dl (normal level of phenylalanine in the blood is 1 mg/dl).
2. *Ferric chloride test:* It is a screening test. Addition of few drops of $FeCl_3$ in patient urine gives leafy green color by interacting with large amount of phenyl ketones which is found in patients urine.
   It is a nonspecific test as certain other compounds like homogentisic acid (in alkaptonuria), also give this test positive.
3. *Guthrie test:* This is a specific test to diagnose PKU.
   Spores of bacillus subtilis need phenylalanine for growth, hence patient suffering from phenylketonuria has excess phenylalanine in the blood which favors the growth of bacillus subtilis.

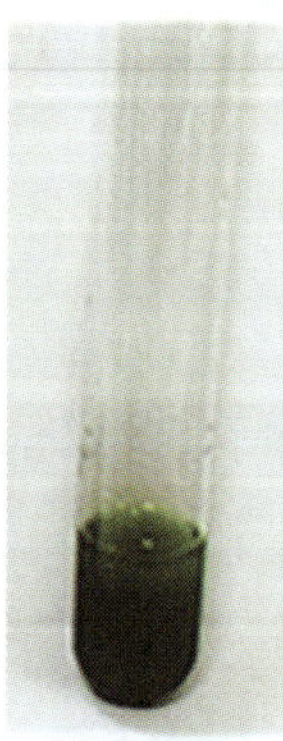

Fig. 19.2: $FeCl_3$ test (green leafy colour)

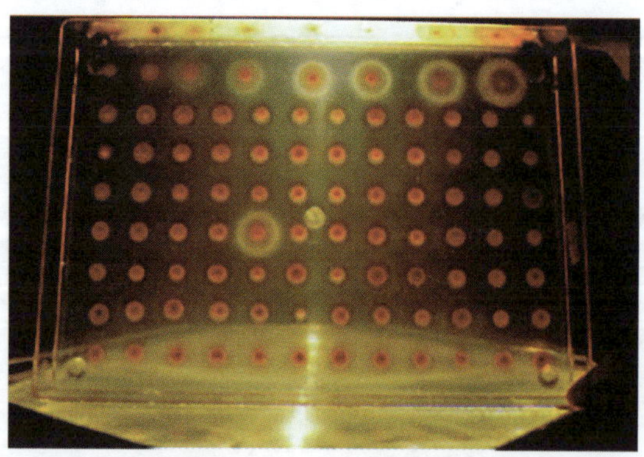

Fig. 19.3: Guthrie test

TYROSINE

Tyrosine is the nonessential glucogenic and ketogenic amino acid. Biologically important compounds produced by tyrosine are:

1. Melanin
2. Catecholamines
3. Thyroid hormone

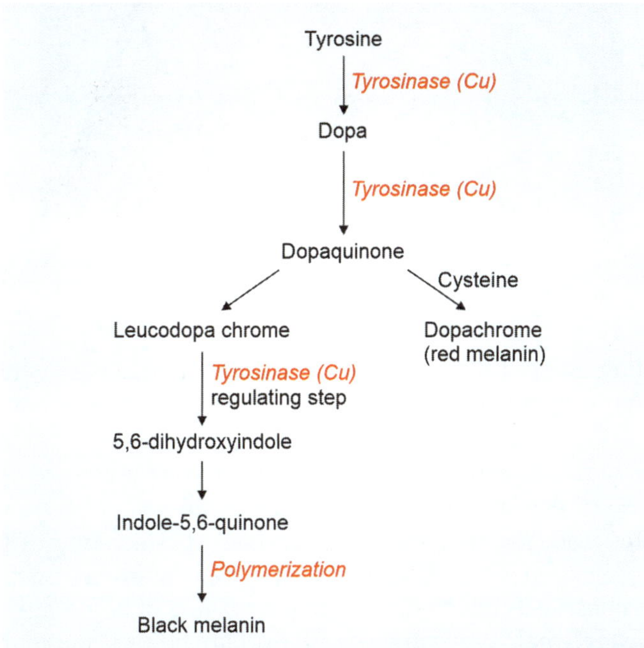

Fig. 19.4: Synthesis of melanin from tyrosine

Key Notes

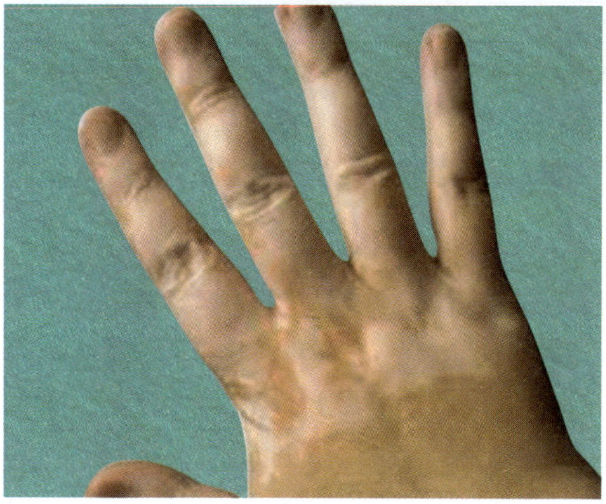

Fig. 19.5: Normal process of melanin production in the skin

Clinical Correlation

- **Albinism:** In this autosomal recessive disorder, there is mutation of tyrosinase gene resulting in absolute lack of synthesis of melanin. Melanin is totally absent from skin and hair which are characteristically white. Incidence is 1:20,000.
- **Leucoderma (vitiligo):** It is an autoimmune disorder, where autoantibodies are developed against melanoblast destroying them. So, that area of skin does not have melanin synthesis.
- **Copper deficiency:** Cu is the cofactor for tyrosinase enzyme. In deficiency of Cu, either because of dietary deficiency or because of defect in Cu absorption from gastrointestinal tract (GIT) (Menkes kinky steely hair syndrome), melanin synthesis gets affected, resulting in graying of hair (flagging of hair in malnutrition and steely hair in **Menkes kinky steely hair syndrome** can be explained this fashion).

Key Notes

Clinical Correlation

- Parkinson's disease:

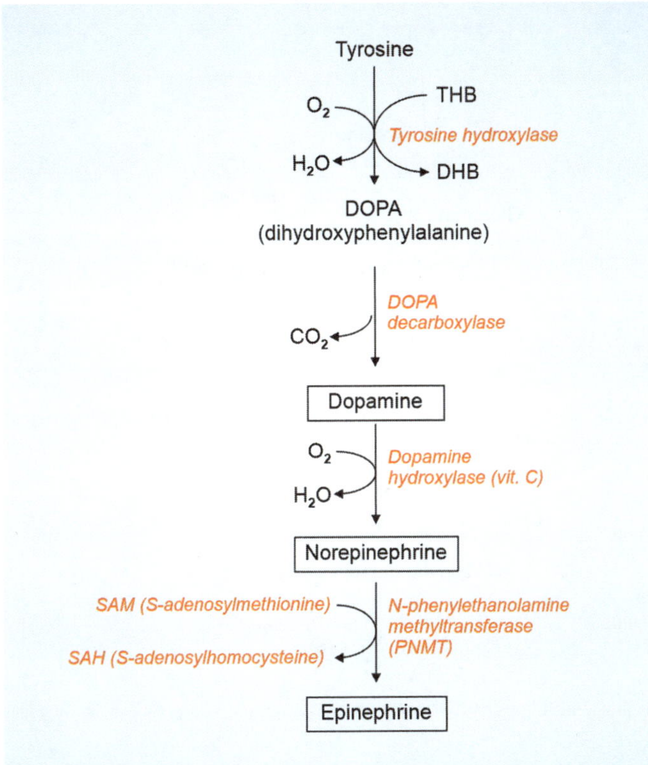

Fig. 19.6: Catecholamine synthesis from tyrosine

Key Notes

Parkinsonism

Tyrosine Catabolism

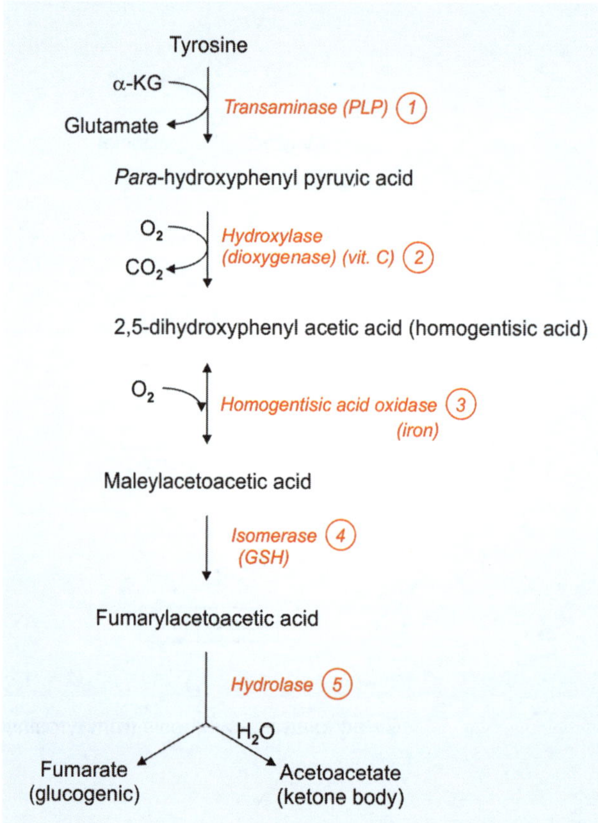

Fig. 19.7: Degradation of tyrosine

Key Notes

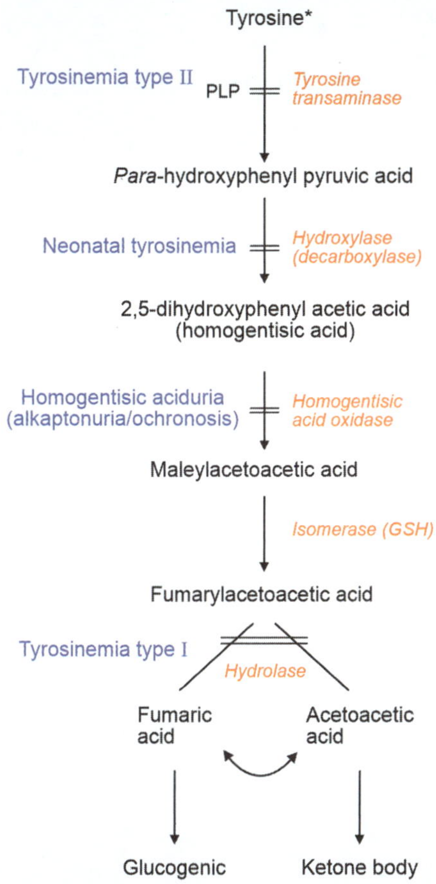

*Tyrosine is both glucogenic (fumaric acid) and ketogenic (acetoacetic acid)

*Incomplete degradation of *para*-hydroxyphenyl pyruvic acid gives rise to tyrosinemia

Fig. 19.8: Clinical disorders associated with tyrosine catabolism

Alkaptonuria

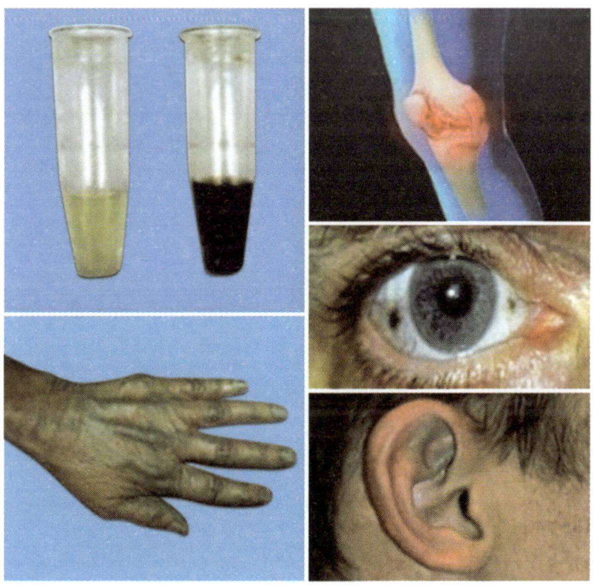

Fig. 19.9: Black pigmentation of skin, sclera, pinnae, joints, black urine

Tryptophan

- Tryptophan is an essential aromatic amino acid.
- Tryptophan is both glucogenic and ketogenic.
- The major pathway where tryptophan is utilized in NAD^+/kynurenine pathway which produces NAD.

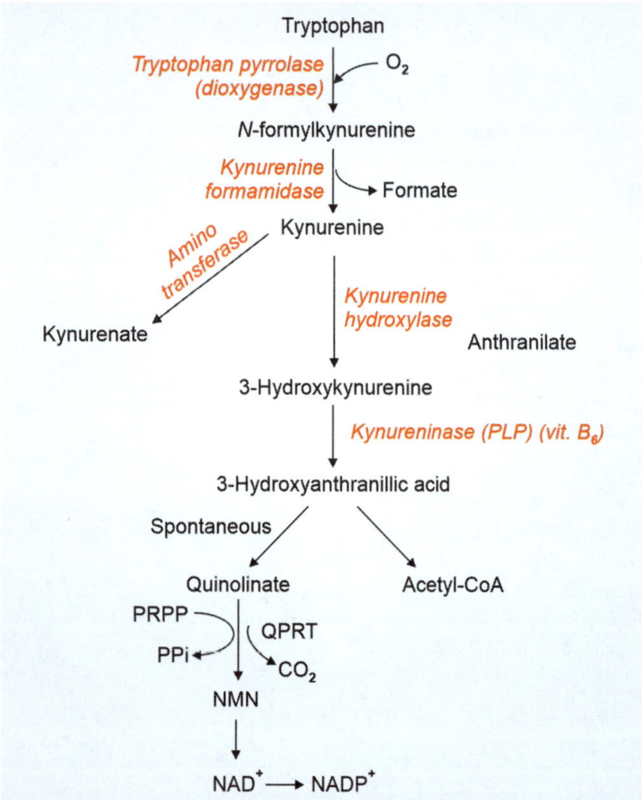

Fig. 19.10: Kynurenine pathway or NAD^+ pathway of tryptophan

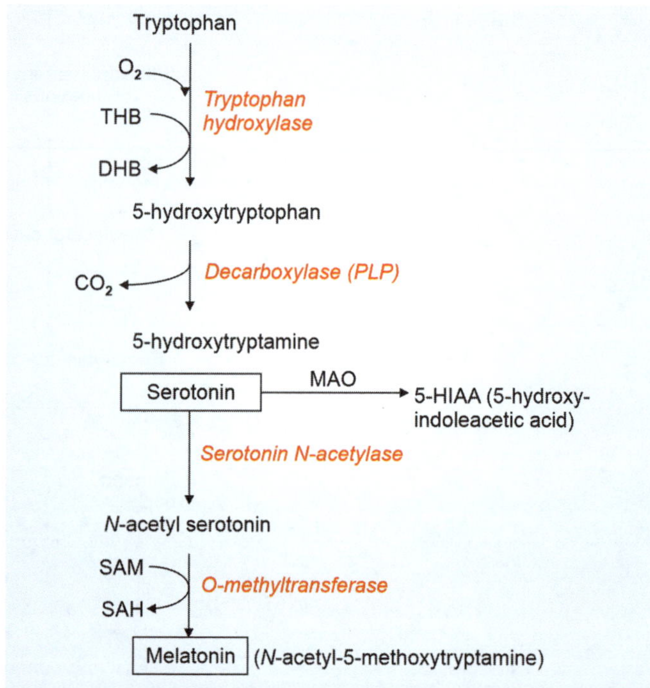

Fig. 19.11: Serotonin/melatonin pathway of tryptophan

Key Notes

20 Electron Transport Chain and Oxidative Phosphorylation

The electron transport chain (ETC) is a set of enzyme complexes where all the components are embedded in the inner mitochondrial membrane (IMM).

ETC is the final common pathway where electron derived from reducing equivalent produced from the oxidation of carbohydrate, lipid and amino acid is finally channelled to an oxygen molecule, which forms water (H_2O)

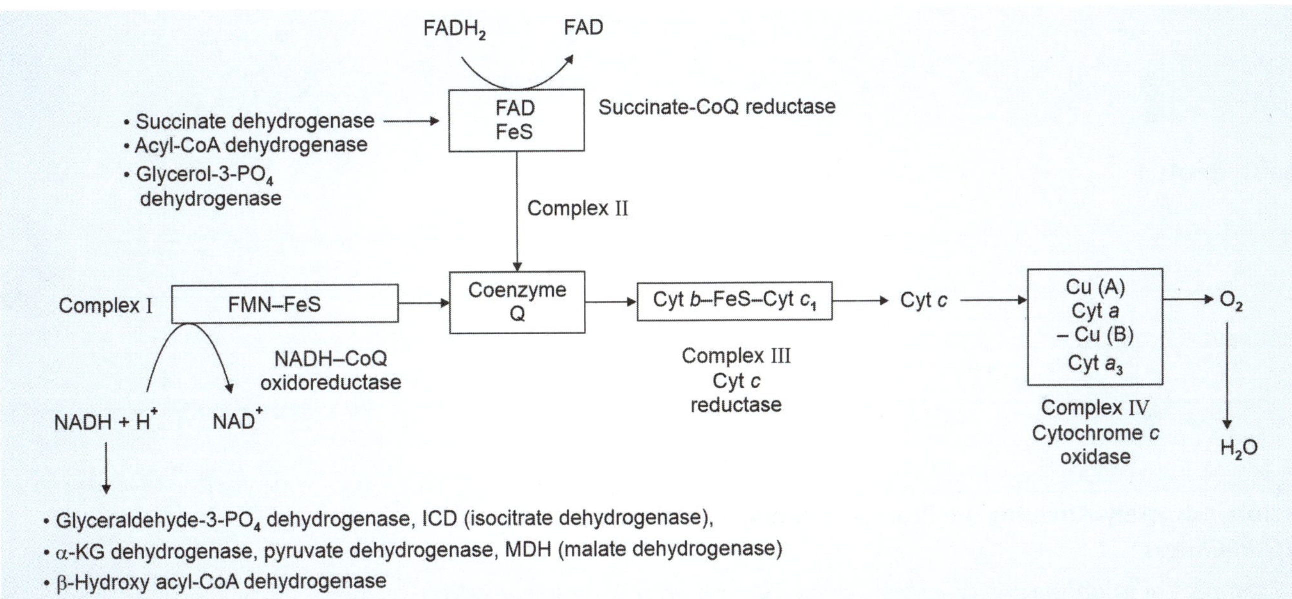

Fig. 20.1: Arrangement of various components in electron transport chain (ETC)

Key Notes

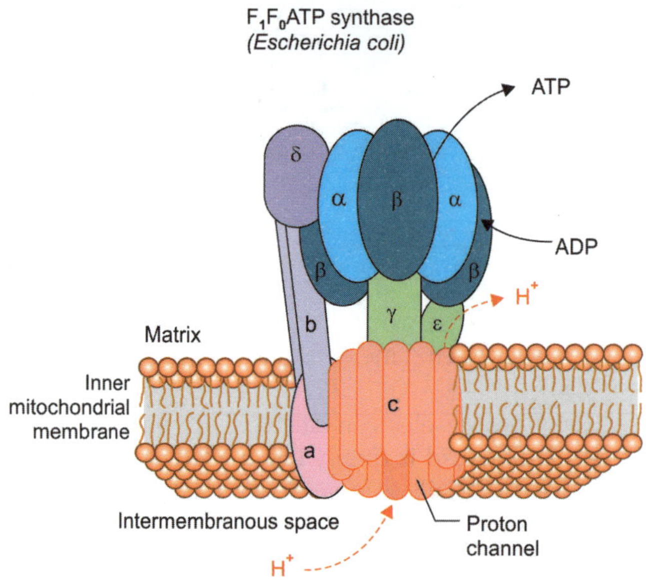

Fig. 20.2: ATP synthase/complex V

Key Notes

Factors Adversely Affecting the Process of Biological Oxidation

ETC Inhibitors

1. *Examples of inhibitors which block e–transmission from complex I to CoQ:*
   a. Rotenone (fish poison)
   b. Piericidin A (antibiotic)
   c. Amytal (barbiturates)
   d. Chlorpromazine (tranquilizer)
   e. Guanethide (hypotensive agent)
2. *Inhibitors which block e–transmission from complex II to coenzyme Q:*
   a. Carboxin
   b. Thenoyltrifluoroacetone (TTFA)
3. *Inhibitors which block the e–transmission within complex III:*
   a. British anti-Lewisite (BAL): Antidote to war gas
   b. Antimycin A
4. *Inhibitors which block e–transmission within complex IV:*
   a. Cyanide
   b. H2S
   c. Carbon monoxide (CO)
   d. Sodium azide

Uncouplers

Uncouplers may be chemical or physiological (natural)

A. Chemical

1. 2,4-dinitrophenol (2,4-DNP)
2. 2,4-dinitrocresol (2,4-DNC)
3. Chloro-carbonyl cyanophenyl hydrazone (CCCP)

B. Physiological (natural)

1. Thermogenin
2. Thyroxine
3. Bilirubin
4. Free fatty acid

Atractyloside: It blocks ATP-ADD antiport on inner membrane of mitochondria, thus prevents entry of ADP into the matrix of mitochondria. ATP synthesis, thus does not take place due to substrate depletion.

Oligomycin: It clamps Fo channel of complex V, thus prevents proton entry back to mitochondrial matrix. This results in no rotation of Y channel and β remains catalytically inactive. This also results in no ATP synthesis.

Key Notes

21

Nucleotide Chemistry and its Clinical Aspects

Components of a nucleotide: Nucleotides are made up of three components:
1. Base
2. Pentose
3. Phosphate

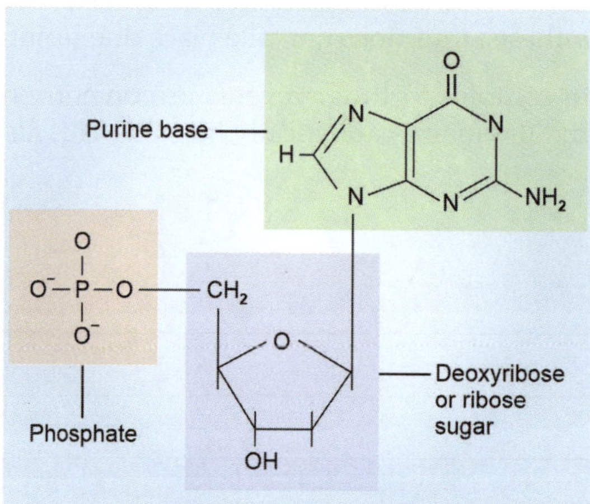

Fig. 21.1: Structure of a typical nucleotide

PURINE NUCLEOTIDE

Biosynthesis of Purine Nucleotide

Three processes contribute to the biosynthesis of purine nucleotides:
1. *De novo* biosynthesis (synthesis from amphibolic intermediates)
2. Salvage pathway (phosphoribosylation of purine)
3. Phosphoribosylation of purine nucleosides (adenosine/guanosine)

1. De novo Biosynthesis (Synthesis from Amphibolic Intermediates)

Contributors for the formation of purine ring during *de novo* biosynthesis are as follows:

Glycine: Contribute C4, C5, N7

Aspartate: Contribute N1

Glutamine: Contribute N3, N9

CO_2: C6

N10-formyl THF: C2

N5 N10-methenyl THF: C8

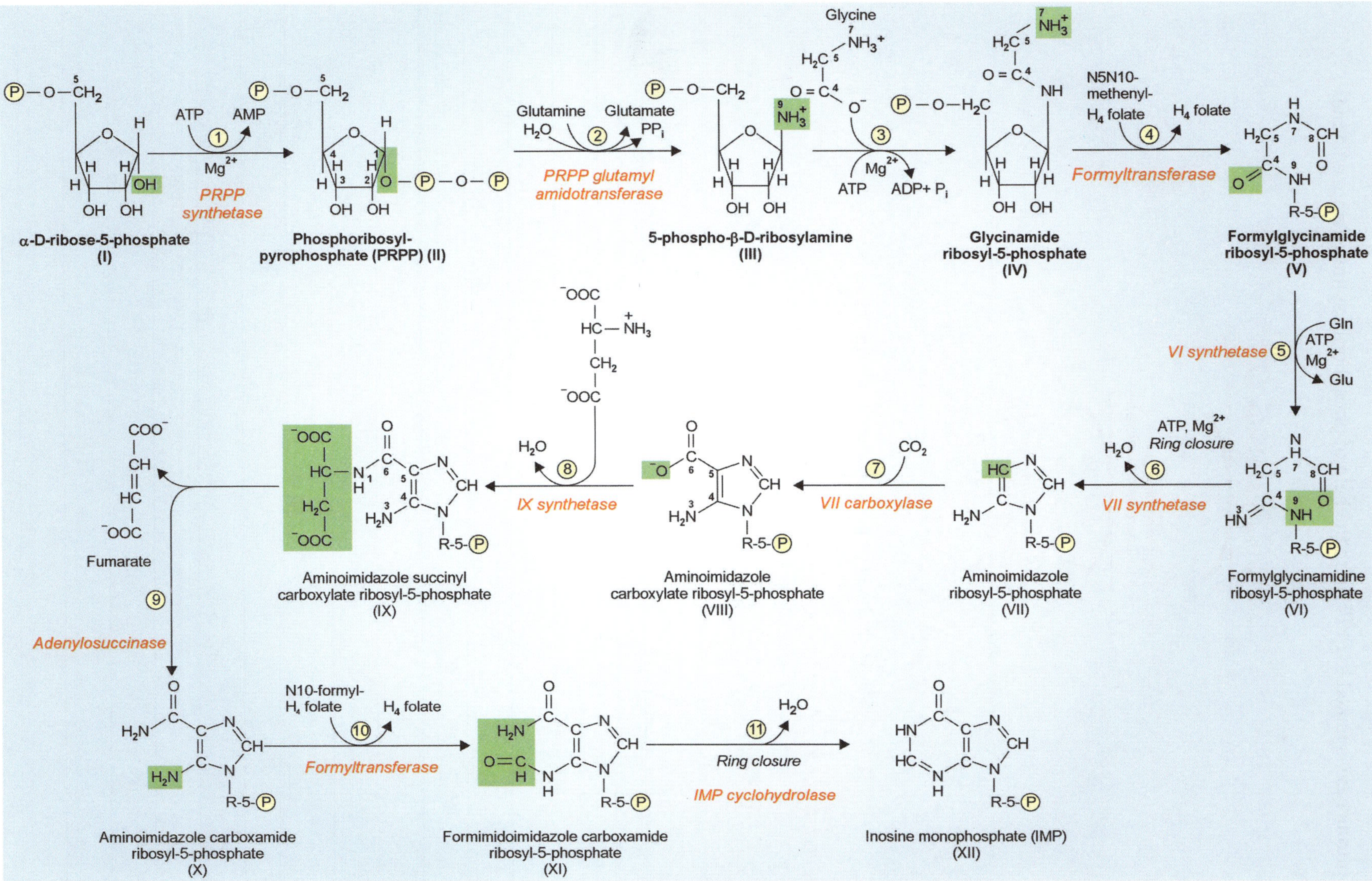

Fig. 21.2: *De novo* biosynthesis of purine nucleotide

2. Salvage Pathway

In this pathway, the purine base is linked to PRPP with the help of phosphoribosyltransferase enzyme.

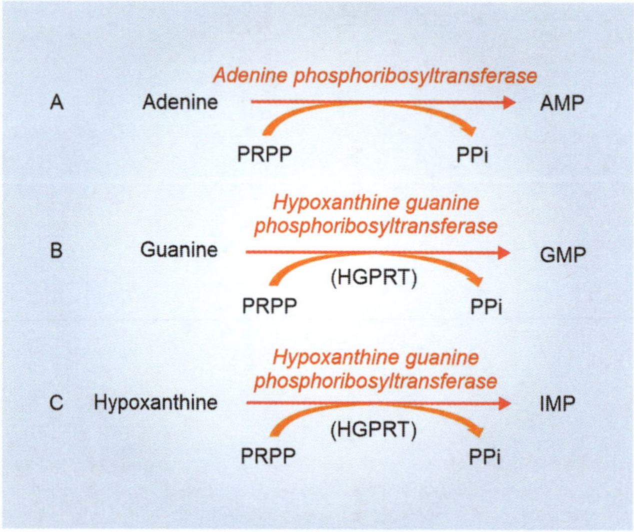

Fig. 21.3: Salvage pathway for purine nucleotide biosynthesis

3. Phosphorylation of Purine Nucleosides (Adenosine/Guanosine)

Key Notes

Catabolism of Purine Nucleosides

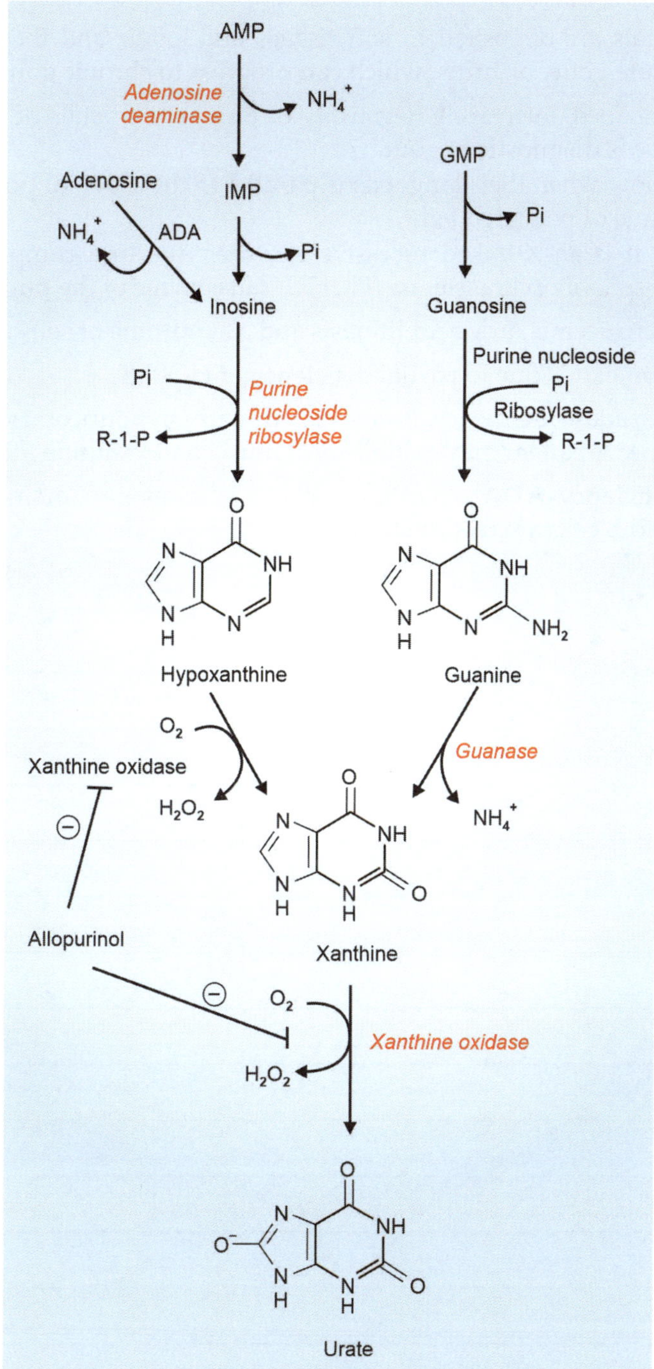

Fig. 21.4: Purine nucleotide catabolism

Key Notes

Clinical Association

Metabolic Disorders of Purine Catabolism

1. **Gout:** Sodium urate crystals are deposited in soft tissues and joints, and they are called tophi, causes an inflammatory reaction, acute gouty arthritis, which can progress to chronic gouty arthritis.
   - Visualization of needle-shaped, intensively negatively birefringent crystals of sodium urate in a joint fluid under a light microscope is diagnostic of gout.
   - The crystals appear yellow when their long axis is parallel to the plane of polarised light, and blue when perpendicular to the plane of polarised light.
2. **Lesch-Nyhan syndrome:** It is an X-linked recessive disorder due to a complete deficiency of the enzyme hypoxanthine-guanine phosphoribosyltransferase 'HGPRT' (an enzyme of the purine salvage pathway).

   It is characterized by hyperuricemia, uric acid lithiasis and a syndrome of self-mutilation.
3. **Kelley-Seegmiller syndrome:** It is due to partial deficiency of HGPRT.
4. **Hypouricemia:** Xanthine oxidase deficiency is associated with hypouricemia and increased excretion of hypoxanthine and xanthine. A patient may exhibit xanthinuria and xanthine lithiasis (stones).
5. **Adenosine deaminase deficiency (ADA):** ADA is associated with severe combined immunodeficiency disease (SCID) in which both T and B cells are dysfunctional.

Key Notes

PYRIMIDINE NUCLEOTIDE

Synthesis of Pyrimidine Nucleotide

- The biosynthesis of pyrimidine nucleotides is mainly through *de novo* biosynthesis.
- This pathway is partly mitochondrial and partly cytosolic.

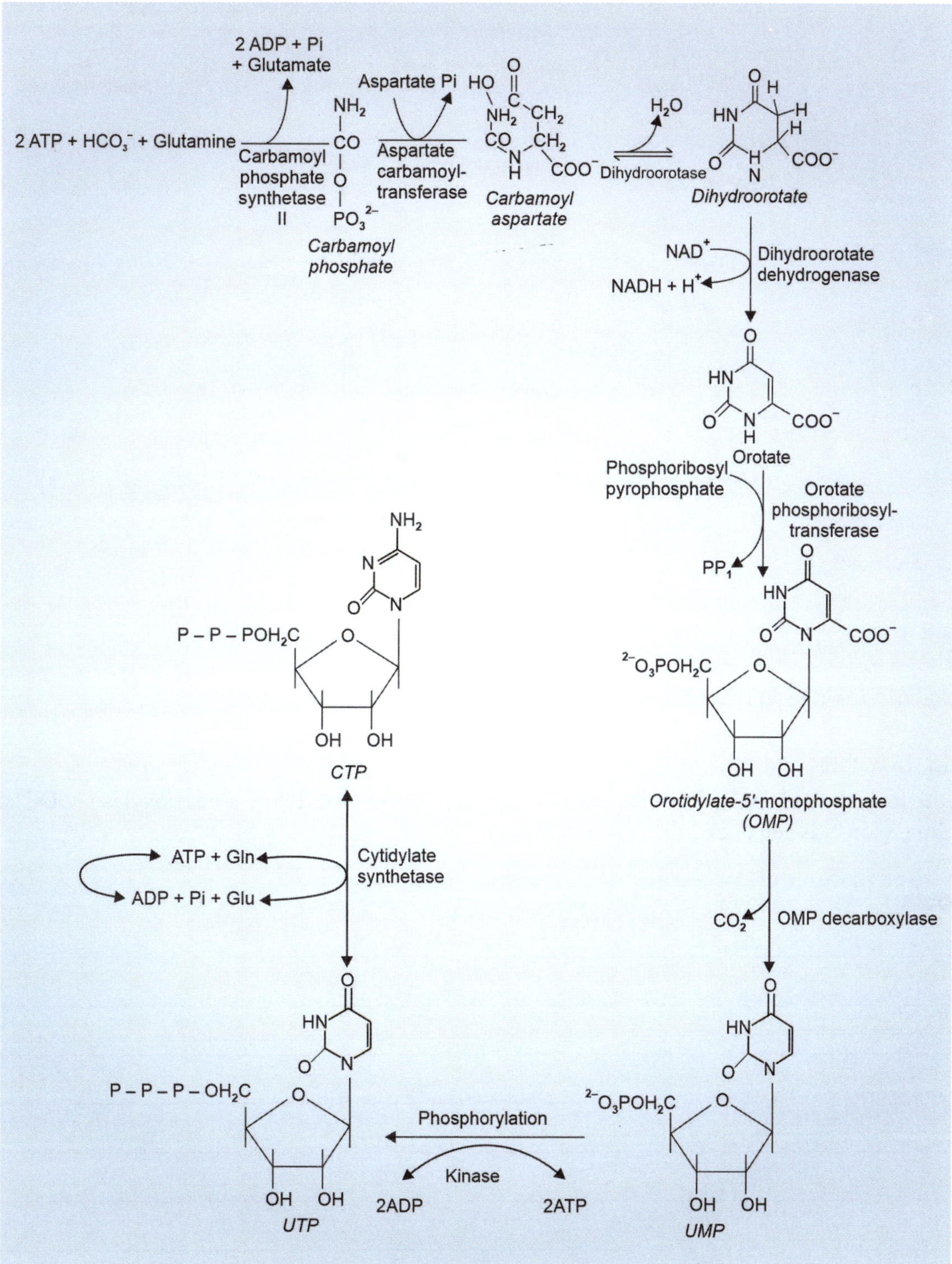

Fig. 21.5: *De novo* biosynthesis of pyrimidine nucleotide

Catabolism of Pyrimidine Nucleotide

The end-products of pyrimidine catabolism are CO_2, NH_3, β-alanine and β-aminoisobutyrate.

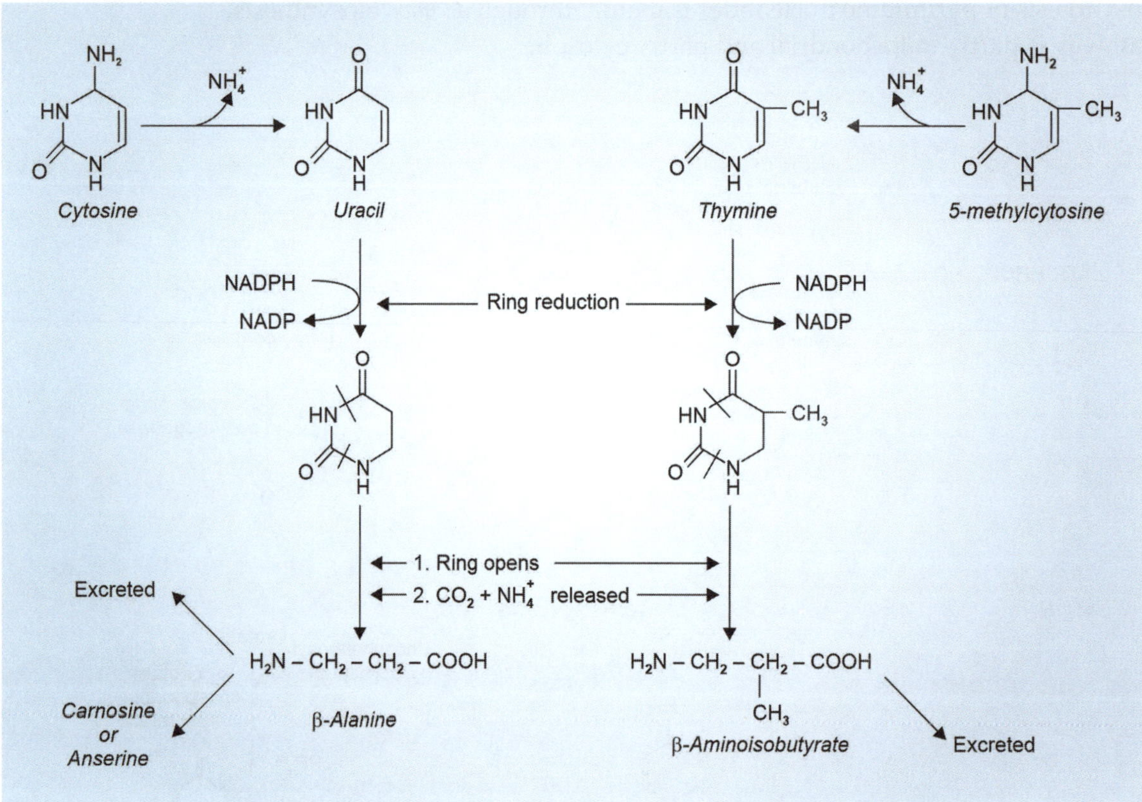

Fig. 21.6: Catabolism of pyrimidine nucleotides

Disorder Associated with Pyrimidine Nucleotide Metabolism

Orotic Aciduria

- It is an autosomal recessive disorder.
- Type I: Due to orotate phosphoribosyltransferase deficiency and orotidylate decarboxylase (ODC) deficiency.
- Type II: Due to orotidylate decarboxylase deficiency.

Key Notes

22 Nucleic Acid (DNA and RNA) Structure

TYPES OF NUCLEIC ACIDS

1. Deoxyribonucleic acid (DNA)
2. Ribonucleic acid (RNA)

Deoxyribonucleic Acid (DNA)

Watson and Crick Model of DNA

Proposed in 1953 by James Watson and Francis Crick.

- It is a double-stranded structure. Each strand possesses polarity and they are arranged in antiparallel direction.
- DNA backbone is made up of phosphodiester bond and bases are perpendicular to the helical axis.
- The two strands of DNA are coiled around a common axis.
- Helix is repeated at interval of 34Å.
- Each helix has 10 base pairs and distance between adjacent bases on a strand is 3.4Å.
- Width of helix is 20Å (2.0 nm).
- The two strands of double-stranded helix are held in place by hydrogen bonds between the purines and pyrimidine bases.
- Adenine pairs with thymine with two hydrogen bonds and guanine pairs with cytosine with the help of three hydrogen bonds ($A = T$, $C \equiv G$).
- Major and minor grooves are present on double helix DNA.

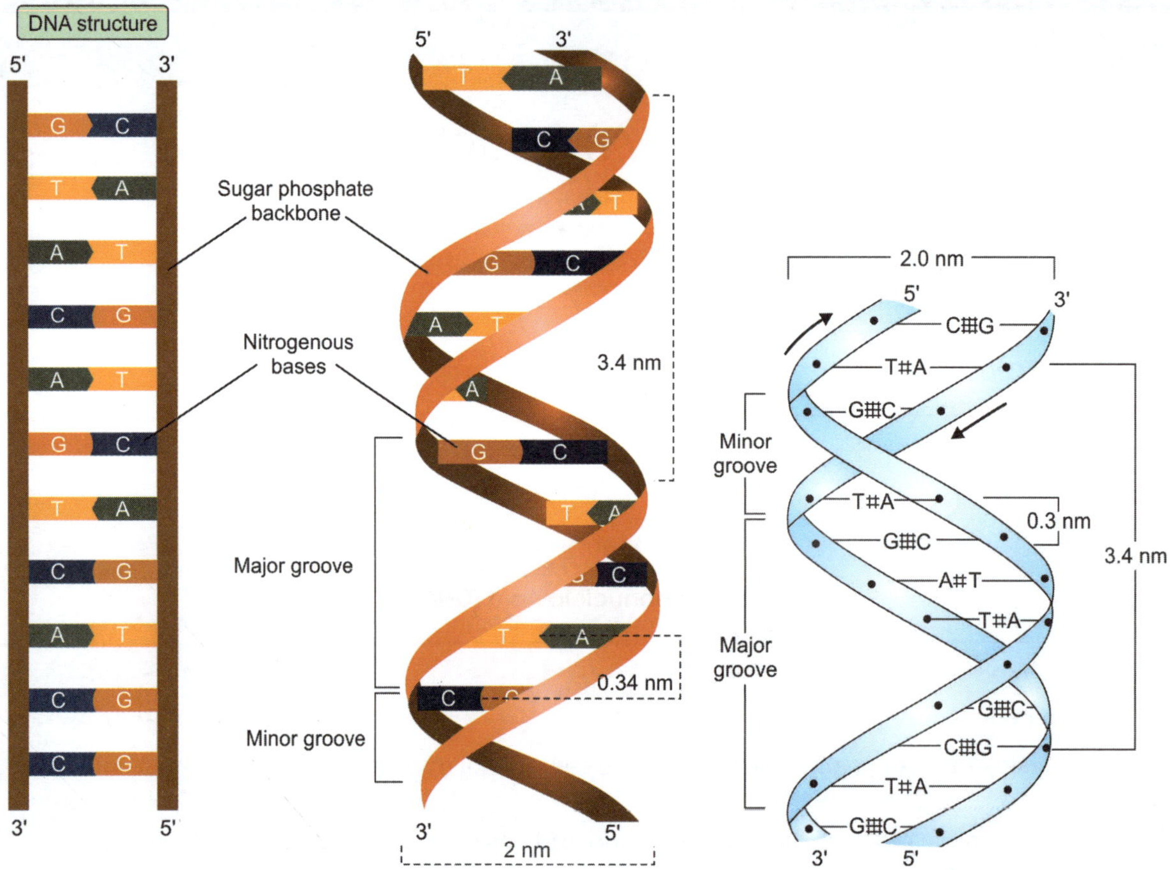

Fig. 22.1: Waston and Crick model of DNA

Key Notes

Nucleosome

- It is a specific of eukaryotic dsDNA and the histone protein octamer.
- Histone proteins are of five types—H1, H2A, H2B, H3, H4.

Key Notes

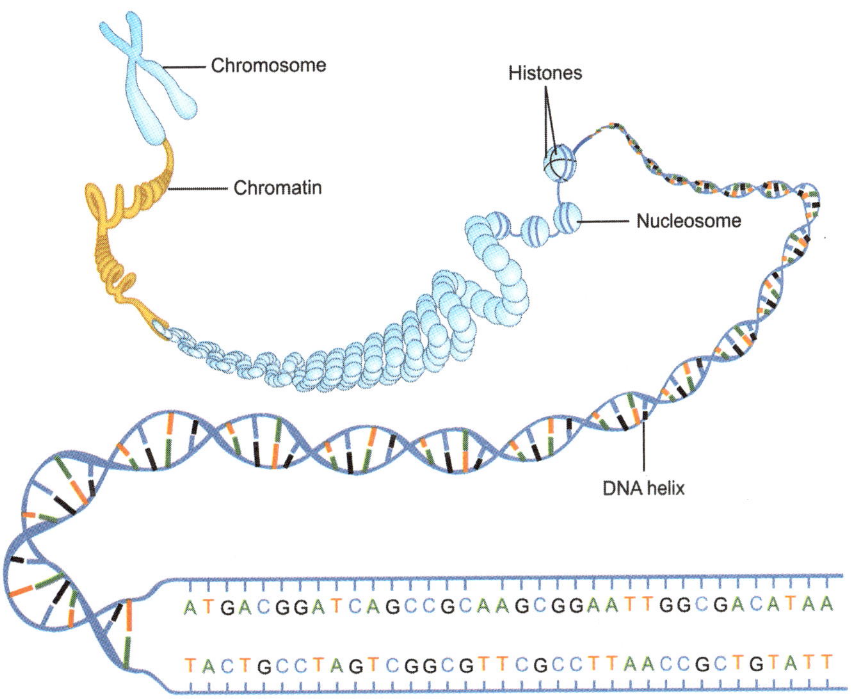

Fig. 22.2: Organization of DNA into chromosome

Ribonucleic Acid (RNA)

Types of RNA in eukaryotes

- Messenger RNA (mRNA)
- Ribosomal RNA (rRNA)
- Transfer RNA (tRNA)
- Small nuclear RNA (snRNA)
- Small nucleolar RNA (SnoRNA)
- Small cytoplasmic RNA (ScRNA)
- Heterogeneous nuclear RNA (hnRNA)
- Small RNA (miRNA and siRNA)

Ribosomal RNA (rRNA)

Ribosomal RNA presents in various ribosomal subunits and helps in the making the body of the ribosome.

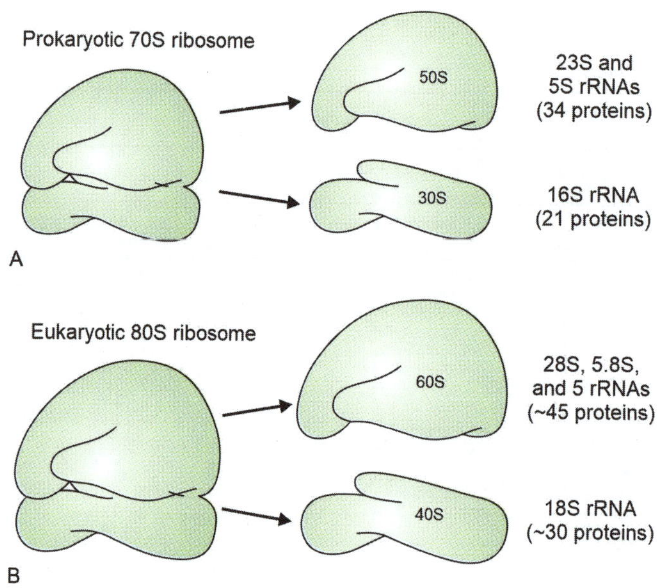

Fig. 22.3A and B: Composition of subunits of eukaryotic and prokaryotic ribosomes

Key Notes

Transfer RNA (tRNA) (Also Called Soluble RNA)

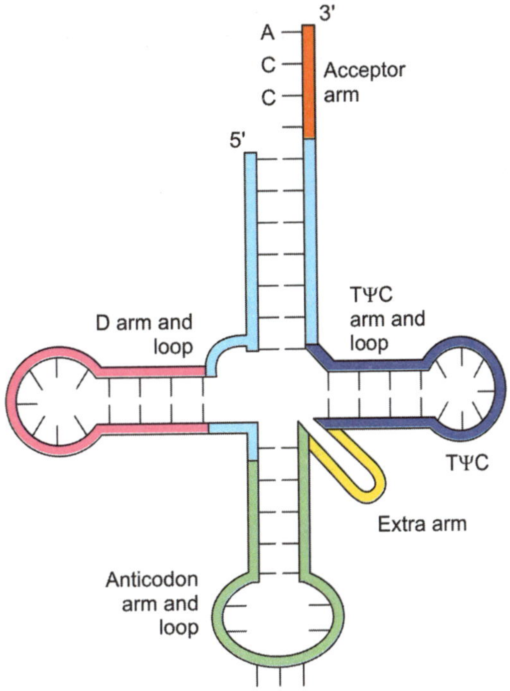

Fig. 22.4: Structure of tRNA

Key Notes

23 DNA Replication in Prokaryotes and Eukaryotes

- DNA replication is also known as DNA synthesis or DNA duplication.
- Whether it is prokaryotic or eukaryotic DNA replication, it is always semiconservative.
- Semiconservative replication means new set of DNA has one parent strand and one daughter strand.

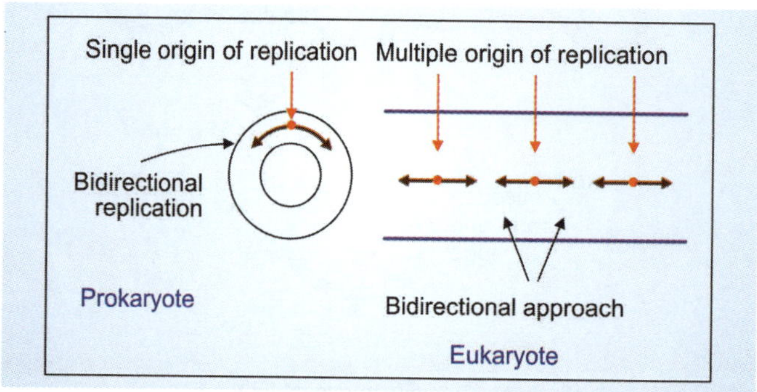

Fig. 23.1: Prokaryotic and eukaryotic DNA replication

Key Notes

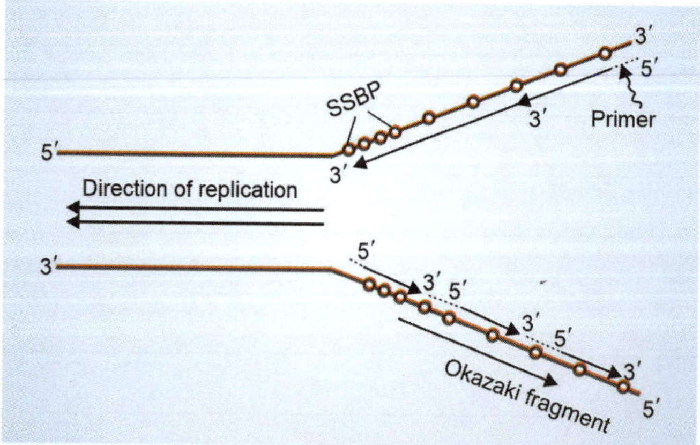

Fig. 23.2: DNA replication

Table 23.1: Enzymes and protein factors needed for DNA replication in prokaryotes

Enzymes/proteins	Role
DNA A protein	Open duplex DNA
DNA B protein	Helicase (unwind)
DNA C protein	Binding of DNA B protein at the origin
DNA G protein	Primase
Single-strand binding protein (SSBP)	Binding of single strand
HU (histone-like)	Stimulates initiation
DNA topoisomerase I	Relieves torsional strain
DNA topoisomerase II (DNA gyrase)	Introduces negative supercoiling

The main enzyme of this phase of DNA replication is DNA polymerase. DNA polymerase is of the following types:

- DNA polymerase I
- DNA polymerase II
- DNA polymerase III

Kornberg discovered DNA polymerase I and named it Kornberg enzyme.

DNA polymerase I has the following activity:

- 5′–3′ polymerase activity
- 3′–5′ exonuclease activity
- 5′–3′ exonuclease activity

DNA polymerase II and III have the following activity:

- 5′–3′ polymerase activity
- 3′–5′ exonuclease activity
- 5′–3′ exonuclease activity is not seen in DNA polymerase II and III

Key Notes

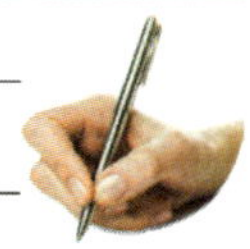

<table>
<tr><th colspan="3">Table 23.2: Comparison of DNA replication of prokaryotes and eukaryotes</th></tr>
<tr><th>Prokaryotes</th><th colspan="2">Eukaryotes</th></tr>
<tr><td>DNA is double-stranded circular molecule</td><td colspan="2">DNA is double-stranded linear molecule open at both of its ends</td></tr>
<tr><td>Origin of replication at 'ori', single origin of replication</td><td colspan="2">Origin of replication at AT rich 'ARS' sequence in yeast, multiple origin of replication</td></tr>
<tr><td>Replication proceeds bidirectionally</td><td colspan="2">Here too, replication proceeds bidirectionally</td></tr>
<tr><td>RNA primer is needed which is approximately 50-nucleotide long</td><td colspan="2">RNA primer is needed which is much small (approximately 9-nucleotide long)</td></tr>
<tr><td>Number of nucleotides in Okazaki fragment is 1000–2000</td><td colspan="2">Number of nucleotides in Okazaki fragment is approximately 200</td></tr>
<tr><td>Rate of replication is faster (500 nucleotides added per second)</td><td colspan="2">Rate of replication is slower (50 nucleotides added per second)</td></tr>
<tr><td rowspan="4">Types of DNA polymerase: I, II, III</td><td colspan="2">DNA polymerase in eukaryotes: a, b, d, e, g</td></tr>
<tr><td>a: Primase activity</td><td>b: Gap filling</td></tr>
<tr><td>d: Lagging</td><td>e: Leading</td></tr>
<tr><td>g: Mitochondrial DNA</td><td></td></tr>
<tr><td>DNA ligase is required and source of energy is NADH</td><td colspan="2">DNA ligase is required and source of energy is ATP</td></tr>
<tr><td>Drugs inhibiting prokaryotic DNA replication are ciprofloxacin and novobiocin</td><td colspan="2">Drugs inhibiting eukaryotic DNA replication are etoposide, adriamycin, camptothecin</td></tr>
<tr><td></td><td colspan="2">RNA primer removal by RNAase H and FEN-1</td></tr>
</table>

Key Notes

Topoisomerase

There are two classes of topoisomerase in *E. coli*:

a. Type I topoisomerase

b. Type II topoisomerase

Telomerase and Telomere

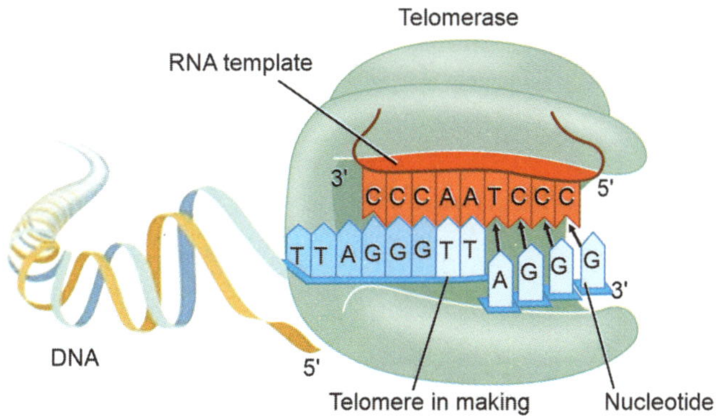

Fig. 23.3: Telomerase

Key Notes

24

DNA Repair Process

Mechanism of DNA Repair

1. Mismatch repair
2. Base-excision repair (BER)
3. Nucleotide excision repair (NER)
4. Double-strand break repair

Key Notes

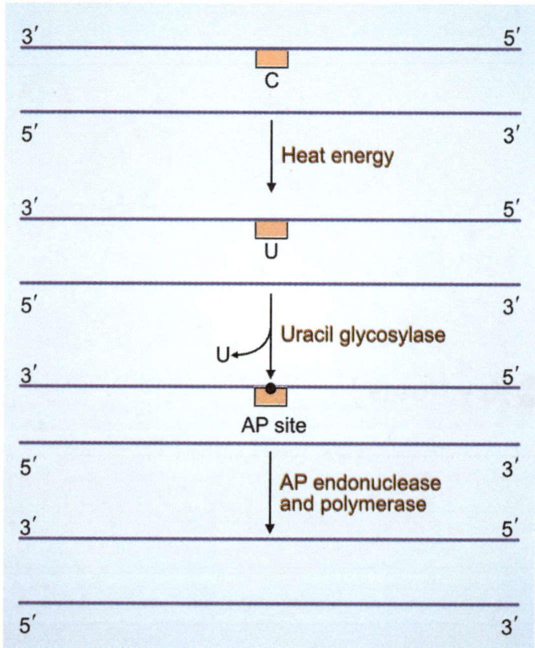

Fig. 24.2: Base-excision repair

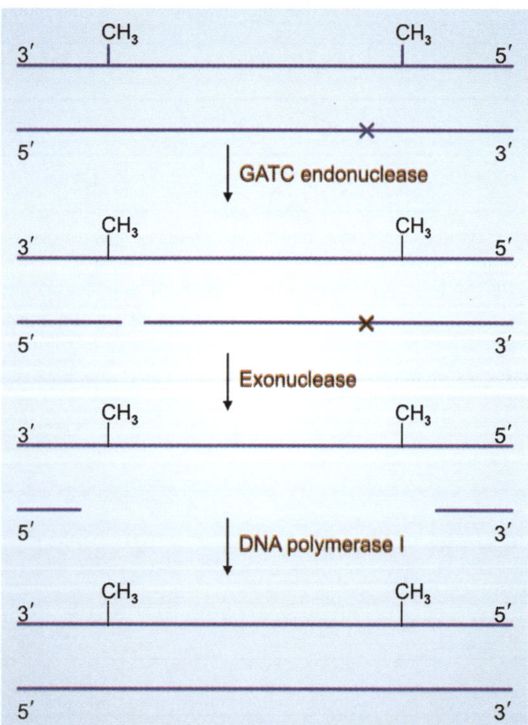

Fig. 24.1: Mismatch repair

Key Notes

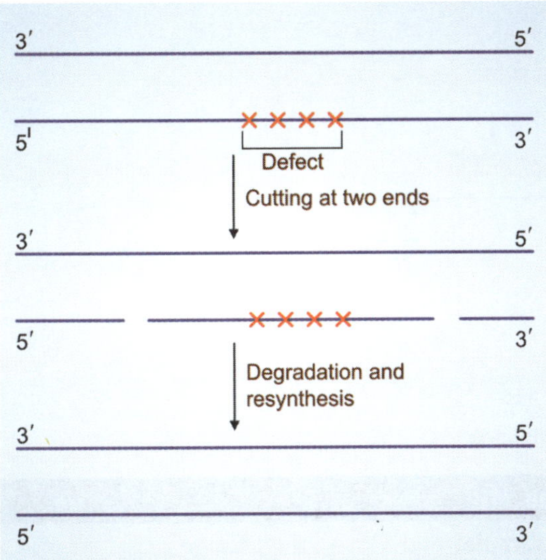

Fig. 24.3: Nucleotide excision repair

Key Notes

Double-strand Break Repair

Double-strand breaks are repaired by one of the two systems:

1. Nonhomologous end-joining repair (NHEJ repair)
2. Homologous recombination repair (HR repair)

Key Notes

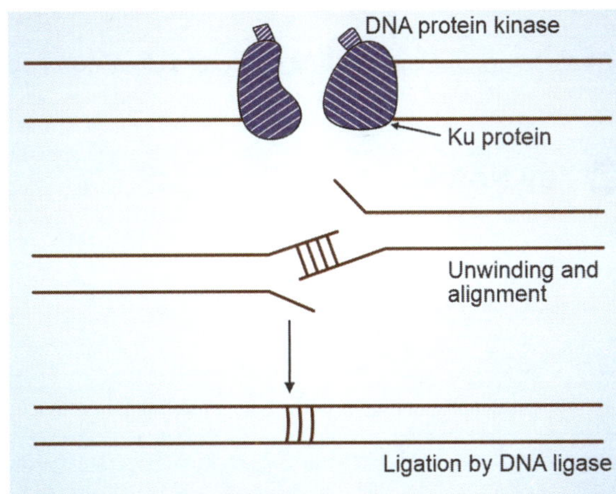

Fig. 24.4: Double-strand break repair

Table 24.1: Defect in DNA repair mechanism and diseases associated with it

Defect in DNA repair mechanism	Diseases associated with it
NER	Xeroderma pigmentosum (XP), trichothiodystrophy (TTD), Cockayne syndrome (Cs)
BER	MUTYH-associated polyposis (MAP)
Mismatch repair	Hereditary nonpolyposis colorectal cancer (HNPCC)
NHEJ repair	Severe combined immunodeficiency disease (SCID)/radiation sensitive SCID (IRS-SCID)
Homologous repair	Bloom syndrome (BS), breast cancer susceptibility 1 and 2 (BRCA-1, BRCA-2), Nijmegen breakage syndrome (NBS), Werner syndrome (WS)

MUTATION

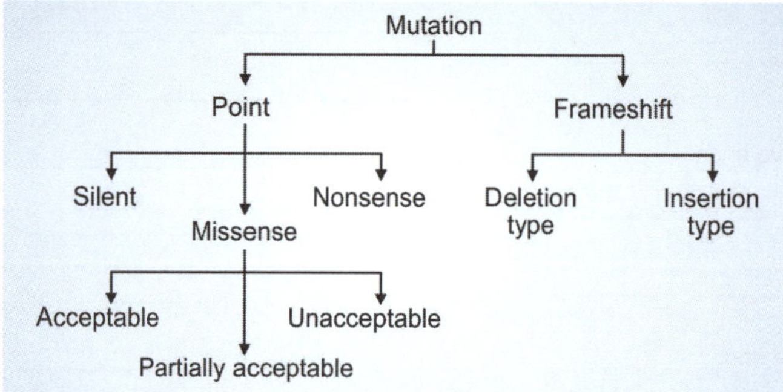

Fig. 24.5: Examples of various mutations

Table 24.2: Point mutations

Type	Effect	Example	Change
Silent	Here, change of codon results in another codon for same amino acid	–	–
	Acceptable	HbA → Hb Hikari	β-Chain 61 Lysine → Asparagine
Missense	Partially acceptable	HbA → HbS	β-Chain 6 Glutamate → Valive
	Unacceptable	HbA → HbM	α-Chain 58 Histidine → Tyrosine
Nonsense	Here, coding is changed to a stop codon after mutation	Boston hemoglobin	–

Key Notes

25 Transcription and Post-Transcriptional Modification

Transcription (RNA Synthesis)

Transcription is the process of synthesis of RNA from the DNA.

Three stages of transcription

- Initiation
- Elongation
- Termination

Eukaryotic Transcription

There are three distinct classes of RNA polymerase enzymes in eukaryotic cells:

1. RNA polymerase I
2. RNA polymerase II
3. RNA polymerase III

Table 25.1: Mammalian RNA polymerases and their products

Form of RNA polymerase	Sensitivity to α-amanitin	Major products	Site
I	Insensitive	rRNA (28S, 18S, 5.8S)	Nucleolus
II	High sensitivity	mRNA, miRNA, snRNA	Nucleus
III	Intermediate	tRNA, 5S rRNA, some snRNA	Nucleus

Key Notes

Eukaryotic Promoters

TATA box

- Most mammalian genes have a TATA box located 15–30 bp upstream from transcript start site (5′-TATAAA-3′), this is also known as Hogness box.
- TATA box binds the 30 KD TATA binding protein (TBP), within turn binds several other proteins called TBP-associated factors (TAFs).
- TBP and TAFs together are known as TFIID. Binding of TFIID to TATA box represents the first step in the formation of transcription complex on the promoter.

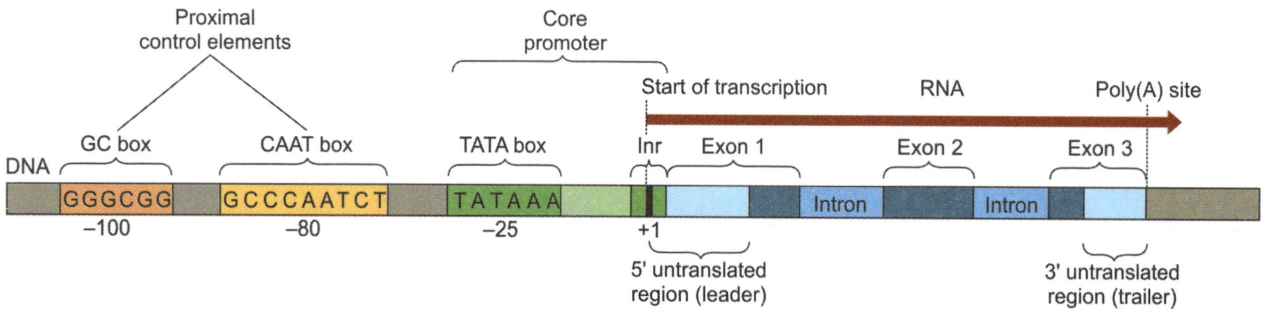

Fig. 25.1: Various promoters on DNA of eukaryotes

The important differences in prokaryotic and eukaryotic transcriptions are enumerated in tabular column

Table 25.2: Differences in prokaryotic and eukaryotic transcription

In prokaryotes	In eukaryotes
• Factors required for transcription:	• Factors required for transcription:
▪ Template strand of DNA	▪ Template strand of DNA
▪ Nucleotides: ATP, GTP, UTP, CTP	▪ Nucleotides: ATP, GTP, UTP, CTP
• RNA polymerase (only one subtype)	▪ RNA polymerase (three types):
	♦ RNA polymerase I
	♦ RNA polymerase II
	♦ RNA polymerase III
• Initiation phase of transcription. Promoter site	▪ Initiation phase of transcription. Promoter site:
▪ –10 region (pribnow box/TATAAT)	♦ –25 region (Hogness box/TATA box)
▪ –35 region: TTGACA	♦ –75 region: CAAT box (GGCAATCT)
▪ Not many initiation factors needed	▪ GC box
▪ Only sigma subunit needed	• Multiple initiation factors needed
• Elongation phase of transcription	
• Phosphodiester bond is formed and RNA synthesis occurs in 5′–3′ direction	• Phosphodiester bond is formed and RNA synthesis occurs in 5′–3′ direction
• No proofreading occurs while elongation	• No proofreading occurs while elongation
• Termination phase of transcription It may be rho factor dependent or rho factor independent	• Termination phase of transcription not well-defined but believed to be similar to mechanism of rho factor independent termination in prokaryotes

Post-transcriptional Modification of Primary Transcript to mRNA

There occur three processes during post-transcriptional modification of hnRNA:

a. 5′-capping
b. Poly(A) tailing
c. Splicing

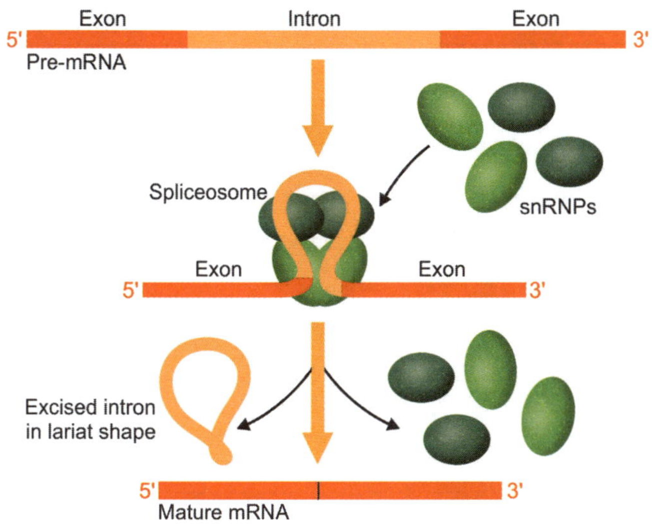

Fig. 25.2: Spliceosomes

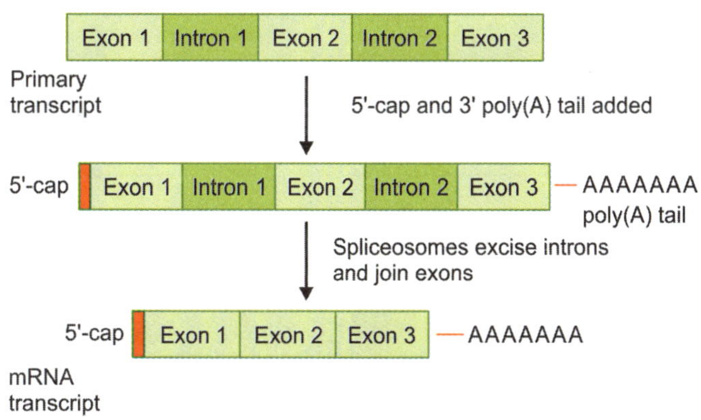

Fig. 25.3: Splicing of primary transcript

Key Notes

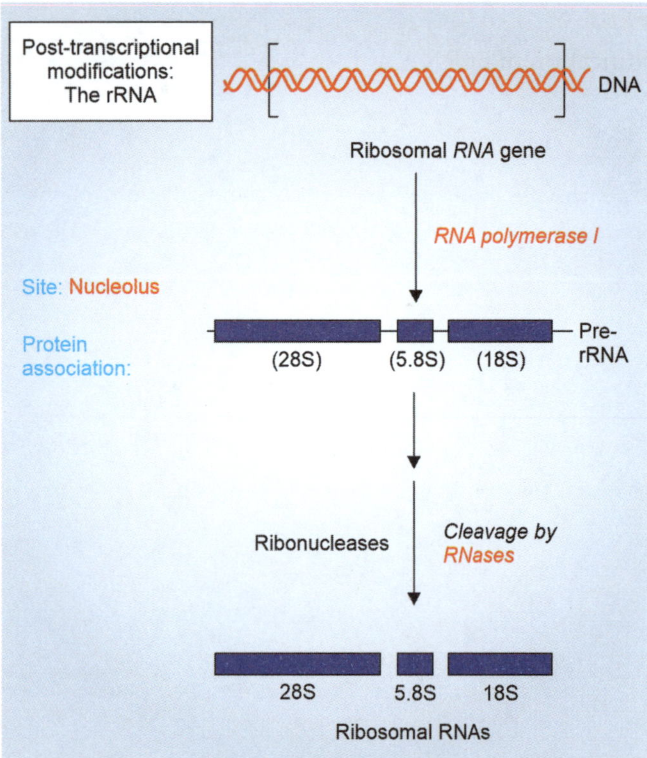

Fig. 25.4: Post-transcriptional modification of rRNA

Key Notes

Key Notes

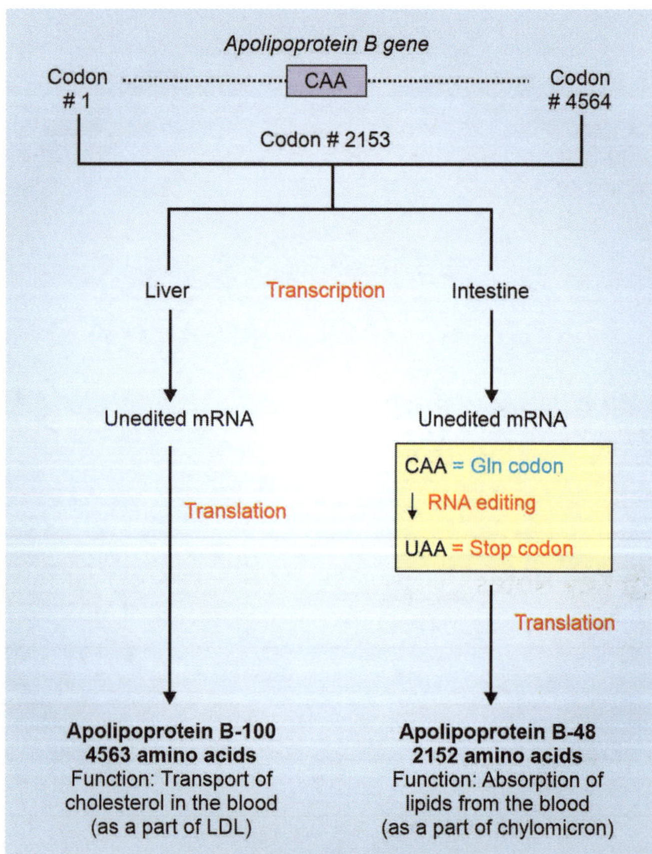

Fig. 25.5: RNA editing (formation of ApoB-100 and ApoB-48 from the same gene by RNA editing phenomenon)

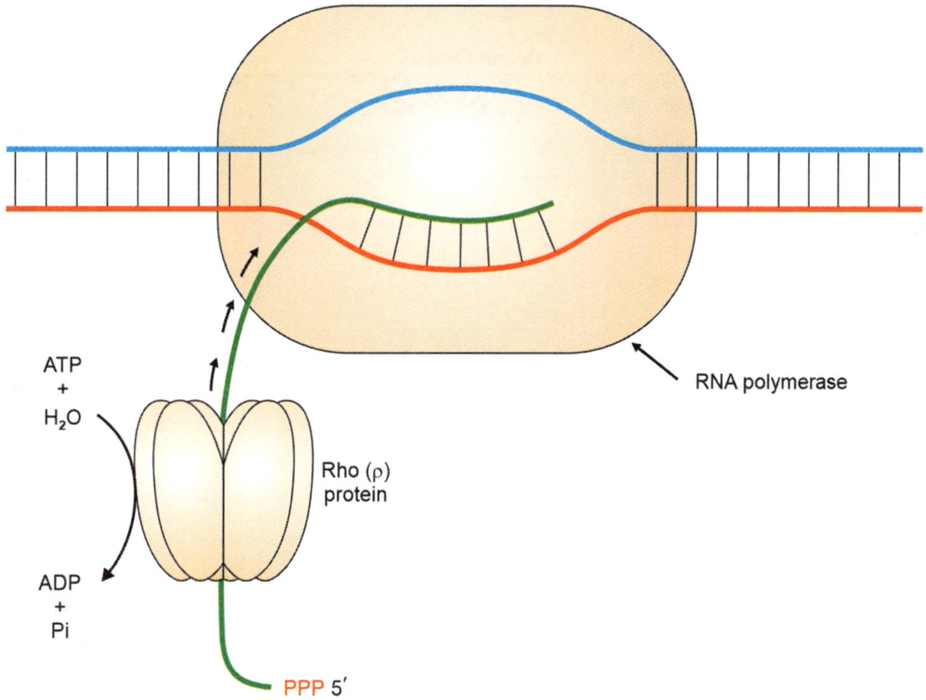

Fig. 25.6: Rho factor dependent termination of prokaryotic transcription

Key Notes

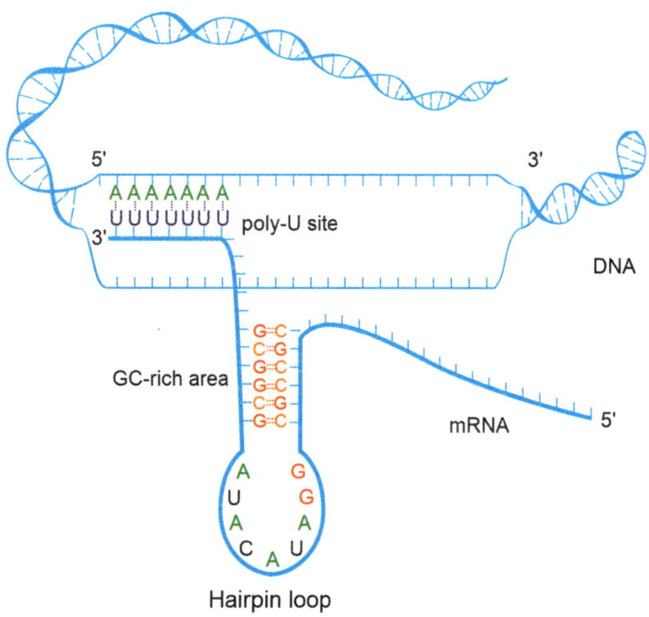

Fig. 25.7: Rho factor independent termination of transcription

Genetic Code

First base	Second base: U	Second base: C	Second base: A	Second base: G	Third base
U	UUU, UUC – Phenylalanine UUA, UUG – Leucine	UCU, UCC, UCA, UCG – Serine	UAU, UAC – Tyrosine UAA Stop codon UAG Stop codon	UGU, UGC – Cysteine UGA Stop codon UGG Tryptophan	U C A G
C	CUU, CUC, CUA, CUG – Leucine	CCU, CCC, CCA, CCG – Proline	CAU, CAC – Histidine CAA, CAG – Glutamine	CGU, CGC, CGA, CGG – Arginine	U C A G
A	AUU, AUC, AUA – Isoleucine AUG Methionine start codon	ACU, ACC, ACA, ACG – Threonine	AGU, AGC – Asparagine AGA, AGG – Lysine	AGU, AGC – Serine AGA, AGG – Arginine	U C A G
G	GUU, GUC, GUA, GUG – Valine	GCU, GCC, GCA, GCG – Alanine	GAU, GAC – Aspartic acid GAA, GAG – Glutamic acid	GGU, GGC, GGA, GGG – Glycine	U C A G

Fig. 25.8: Genetic code

Key Notes

26 Translation

Translation can be divided into three phases:

1. Initiation
2. Elongation
3. Termination

INITIATION

- In this phase of translation, the formation of an 80S initiation complex occurs.
- 80S initiation complex is the arrangement, where protein synthesis takes place during the translation process.

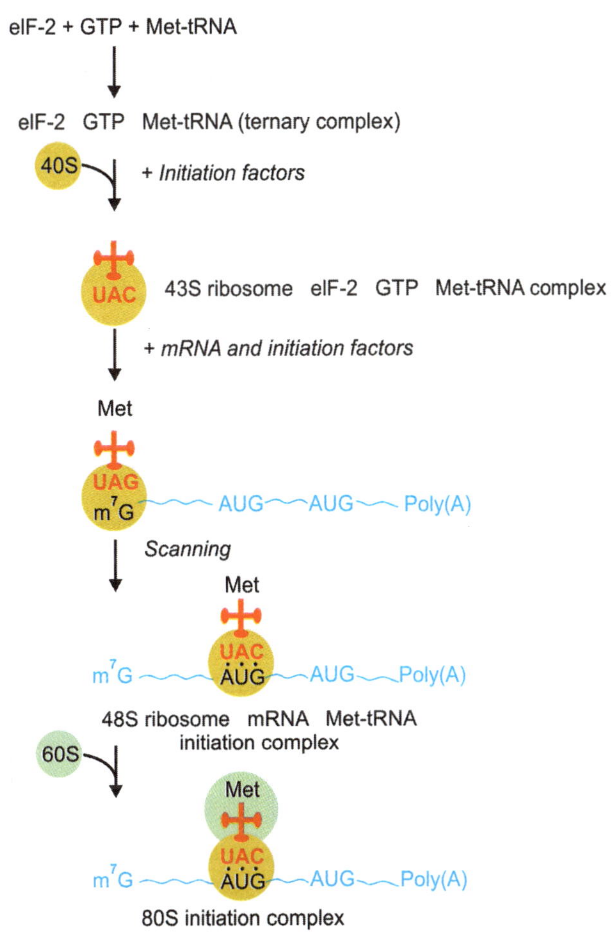

Fig. 26.1: Protein synthesis (formation of 80S initiation complex)

ELONGATION

- In this phase, protein synthesis exists where amino acids are linked through peptide linkage.
- Peptidyl transferase is the ribozyme which plays a key role in translation.

Elongation (translation)

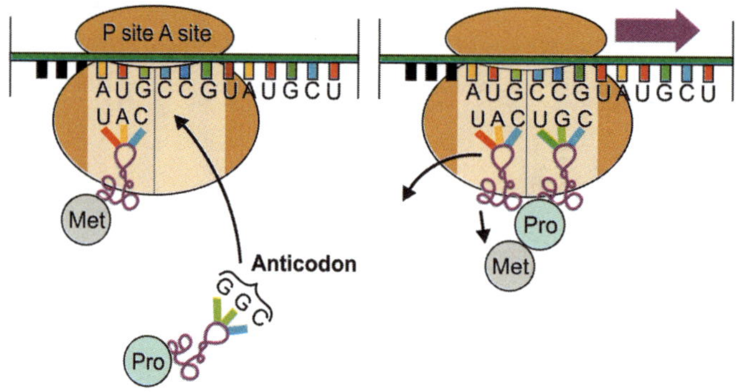

Fig. 26.2: Elongation of polypeptide

TERMINATION

Termination of protein synthesis occurs when either UAA, UAG or UGA is encountered at the A site of the ribosome.

Key Notes

Lac Operon Model

Jacob and Monod, in 1961, described the *lac* operon model. In this model, they explained the regulation of lactose metabolism by an induction or derepression process.

Key Points

- *Repressor protein binds operator region and represses the gene.*
- *Allolactose binds repressor protein and destroys it.*
- *CAP-cAMP binds CAP-cAMP binding site and enhances the ongoing transcription of the gene.*

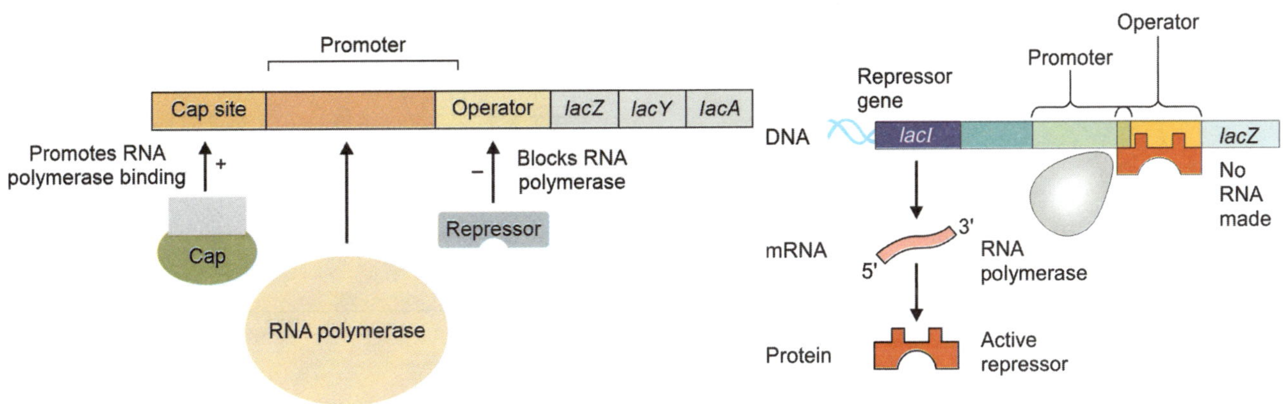

Fig. 27.1: Lac operon model

Key Notes

Section G
Genetic Technologies

28

Recombinant DNA Technology

The process whereby a gene or a DNA fragment of one species is transferred to the DNA of another species is known as recombinant DNA technology or genetic engineering.

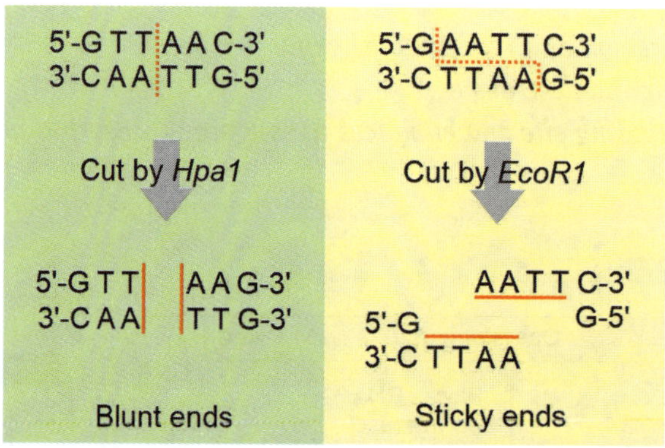

Fig. 28.1: Blunt and sticky ends of DNA produced by action of restriction endonuclease

> ***Key Note***
> ***Restriction Enzyme***
> - This enzyme was first isolated in 1970 by Hamilton Smith who named it beta-Hind-1.
> - These enzymes have tendency to recognise certain palindromic sequences in the DNA, i.e. the sequence which has twofold rotational symmetry.
> - Palindromic sequence is also called inverted repeat. It is a segment of double-stranded DNA, where nucleotide sequence is same in 5′–3′ direction on both the strands.
> - Generally, the size of palindromic sequence is 4–7 bp long.

Vectors for Preparation of Chimeric DNA Molecule

Types of vectors which can be used for the preparation of chimeric DNA

1. Plasmids
2. Bacteriophages, e.g. λ-phage
3. Cosmids
4. Bacterial artificial chromosome (BAC)
5. Yeast artificial chromosome (YAC)
6. P1 vectors

Table 28.1: Cloning capacities of common cloning vectors	
Vector	**DNA insert size (kb)**
Plasmid pBR322	0.01–10
λ Charon 4A	10–20
Cosmids	35–50
Bacterial artificial chromosome (BAC) P1 vector	50–250
Yeast artificial chromosome (YAC)	500–3000

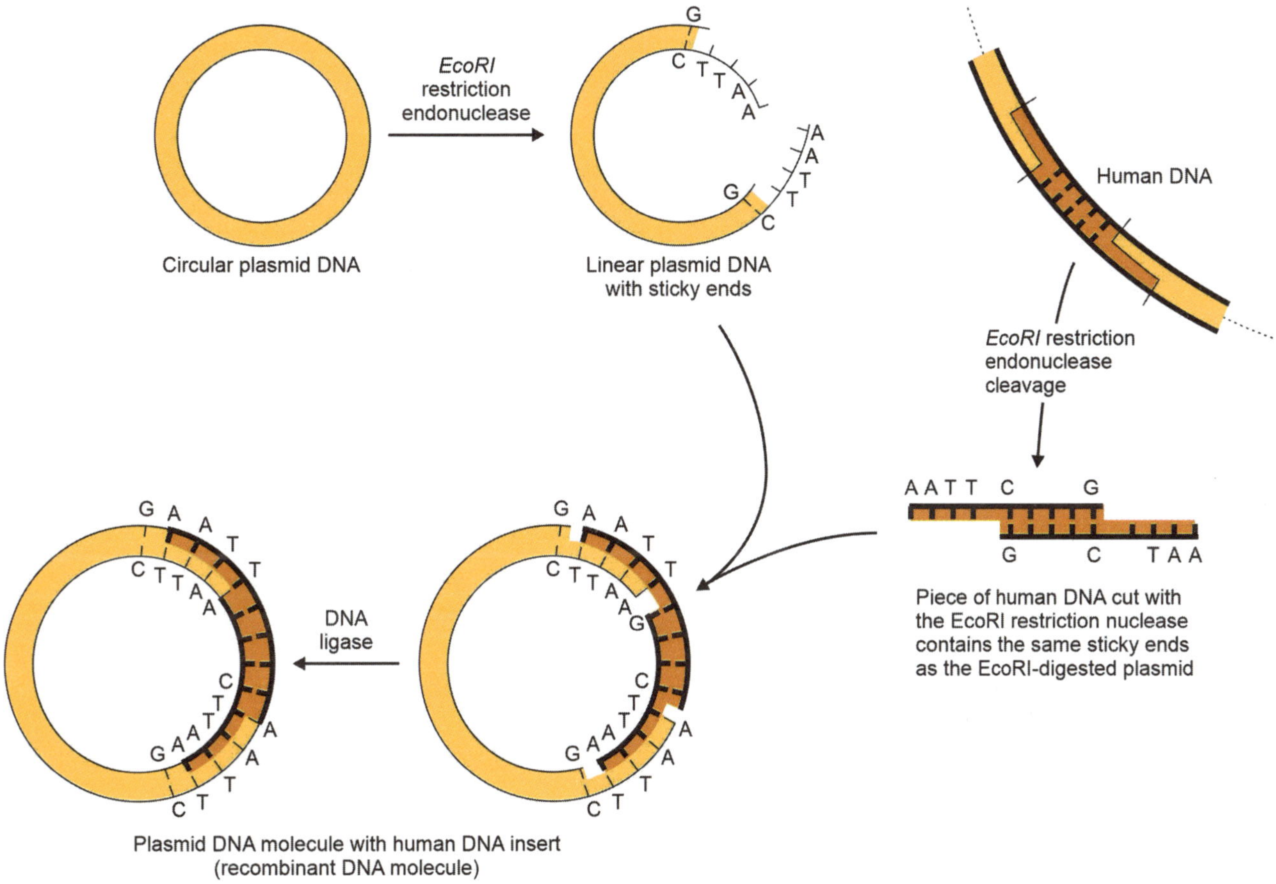

Fig. 28.2: Recombinant DNA technology and formation of chimeric vector

Key Notes

GENE THERAPY

It is the process by which a defective gene is either repaired or replaced by a normal gene to produce the normal functioning gene.

Accordingly, gene therapy may be done in any of the following approaches:

- Gene replacement
- Gene correction
- Gene augmentation

Key Notes

29

Blotting Techniques

Southern Blotting Technique

The following steps are involved in this technique:

- Extraction of the genomic DNA from a cell.
- The action of a restriction enzyme to convert it into a mixture of DNA fragments.
- Electrophoretic separation of DNA fragments on agarose or polyacrylamide gel. DNA, being negatively charged, migrates toward the anode; smaller fragments move the most rapidly.
- Denaturation of DNA by exposure to mild alkali (0.5 N NaOH).
- Transfer of DNA fragment to nitrocellulose or nylon paper, resulting in a replica of the pattern on the gel, by the blotting technique (either manual or electrical blotting).
- Fixation: The transferred DNA fragment is bound to the paper by exposure to heat at 80°C for 1 hour.
- Hybridization of the probe: Nitrocellulose replica is soaked in the neutral solution of the probe at a suitable temperature to allow hybridization of the probe to its complementary sequence.
- Washing and probe identification: After thorough washing to remove excess unbound probe, the paper is exposed to X-ray.

Key Notes

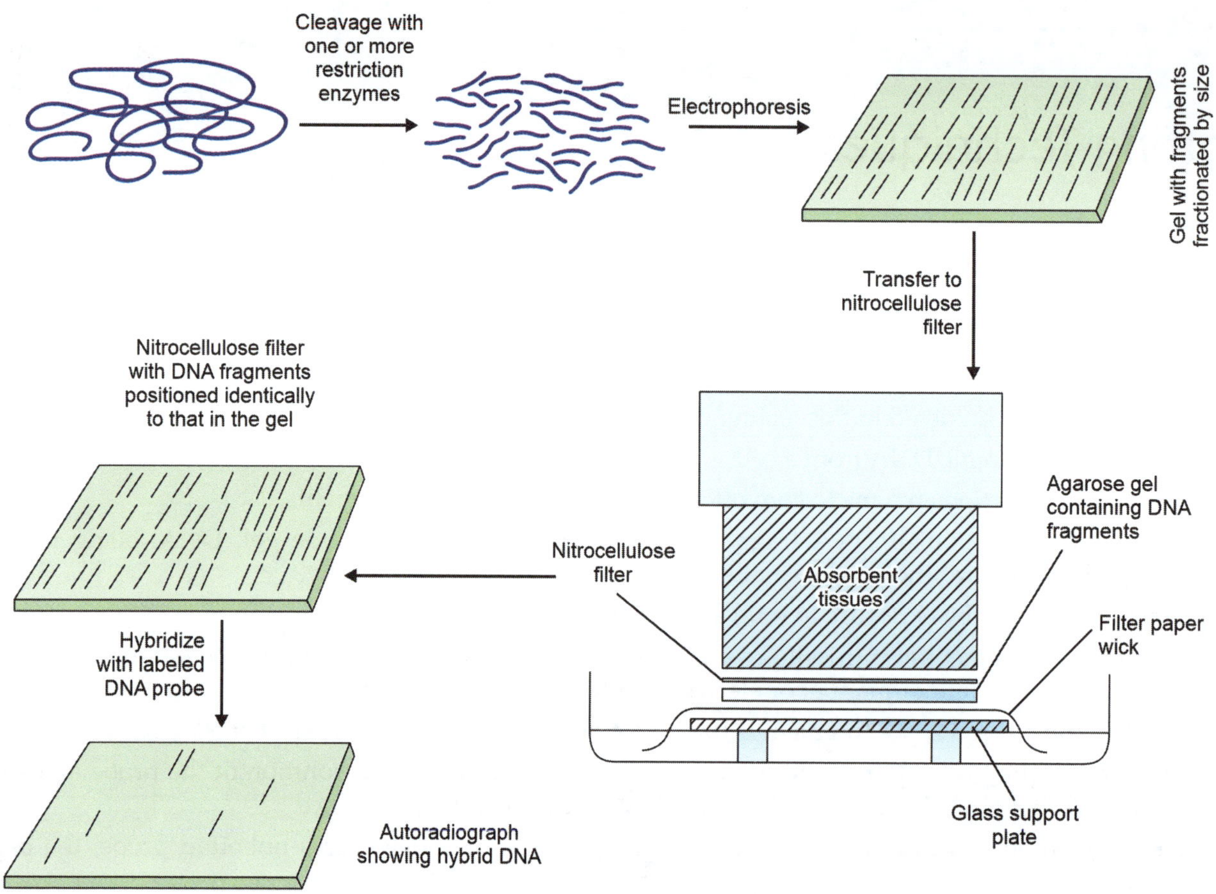

Fig. 29.1: Steps of Southern blot

Key Notes

30

Polymerase Chain Reaction

POLYMERASE CHAIN REACTION (PCR)

The following steps are involved in each cyclical reaction:

a. **Denaturation:** Double-stranded DNA is melted (separated) using heat at 95°C for 15 seconds.

b. **Elongation annealing:** Primer is annealed by reducing the temperature to 50°C for 2 minutes.

c. **Extension:** Taq polymerase (derived from *Thermus aquaticus*) is used to polymerize the DNA at the temperature of 72°C for a variable number of minutes (this duration depends upon the length of the target sequence).

Key Notes

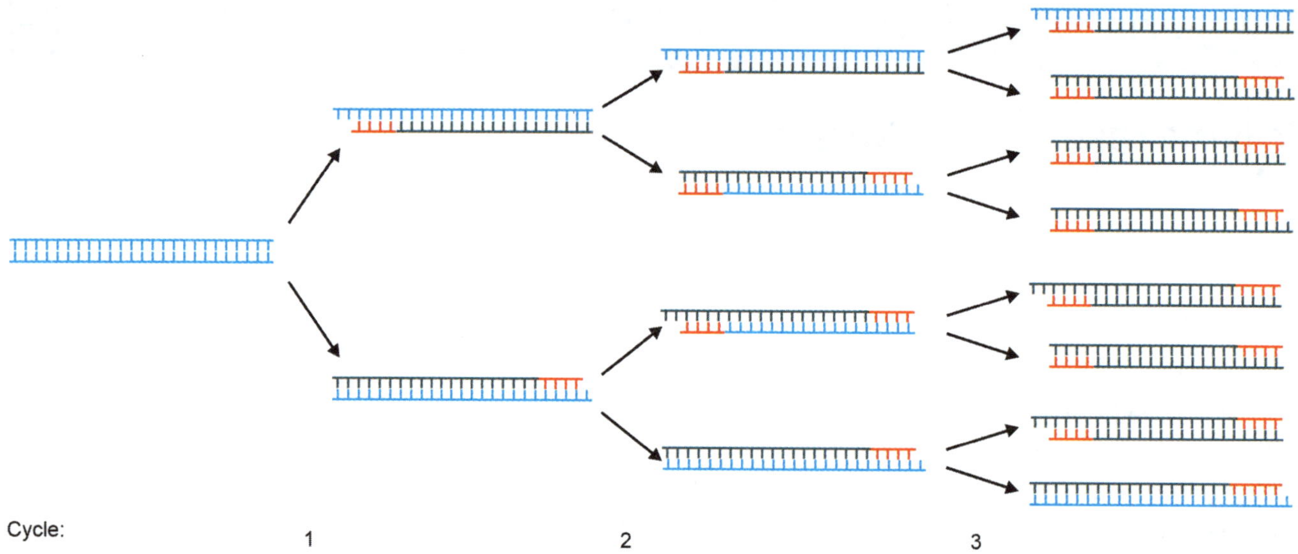

Fig. 30.1: Polymerase chain reaction

Application of PCR

a. In forensic medicine (DNA received from the crime scene is amplified by PCR and is studied).

b. To detect infectious agents (early diagnosis of tuberculosis, HIV and CMV).

c. To make prenatal genetic diagnosis (to amplify the fetal genetic material received from amniocentesis).

d. In the diagnosis of genetic disorders like sickle cell anemia, β-thalassemia and cystic fibrosis.

e. To study evolution, using DNA from archeological samples (fossil study).

Key Notes

31 Restriction Fragment Length Polymorphism

Restriction Fragment Length Polymorphism (RFLP)

An inherited difference in the pattern of restriction enzyme digestion is known as a restriction fragment length polymorphism, or RFLP.

The principle of this technique is polymorphism.

Polymorphism

Detectable, acceptable, inherited or acquired change in the sequence of the nucleotide in the DNA of different individuals is known as polymorphism.

Polymorphism is of two types:

1. Single base change in the DNA (SNP)
2. Variable number of tandem repeats (VNTR)

Key Notes

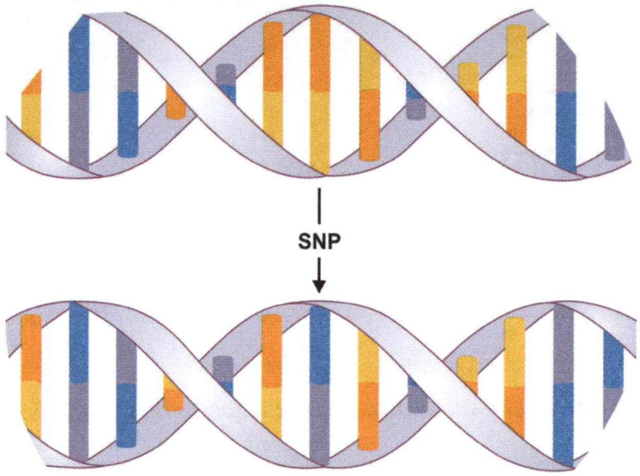

Fig. 31.1: Single nucleotide polymorphism (SNP)

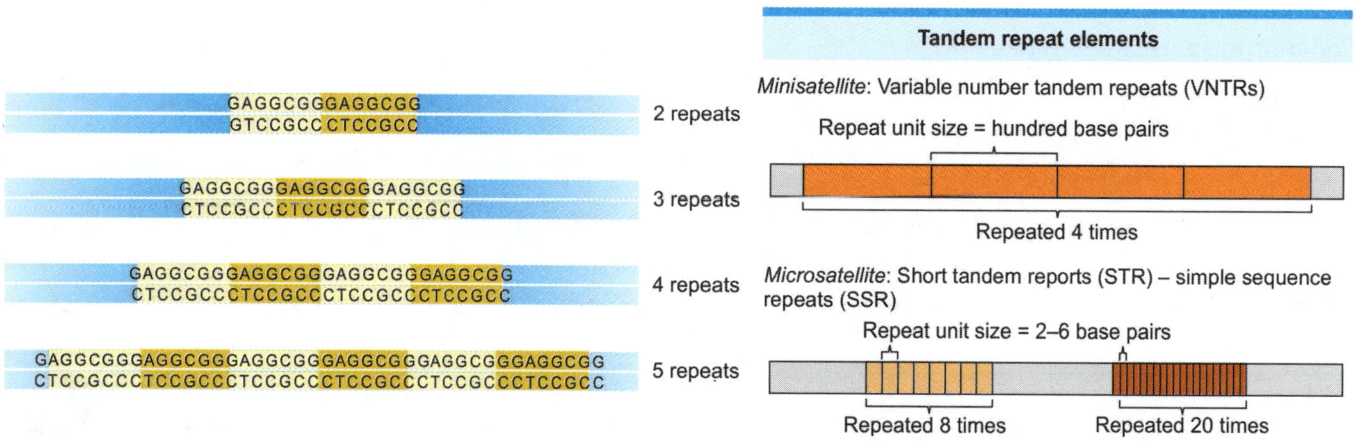

Fig. 31.2: Variable number of tandem repeats (VNTRs)

Key Notes

32

Heme Metabolism

Heme proteins are a group of specialized proteins which have heme as the tightly bound prosthetic group.

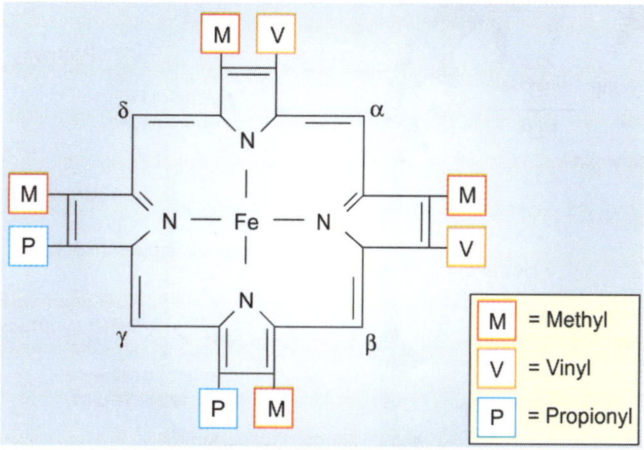

Fig. 32.1: Structure of heme: Tetrapyrrole ring of heme with iron in the center

Examples of heme proteins are

- Hemoglobin
- Myoglobin
- Cytochrome C
- Cytochrome P450
- Catalase
- Peroxidase
- Tryptophan pyrrolase
- Nitric oxide synthase
- Guanylyl cyclase

Key Notes

Synthesis of Heme

- Synthesis of heme takes place in two organs: Bone marrow and liver
- 85% of heme synthesis occurs in bone marrow cells, and 15% in the liver.
- The complex heme molecule is synthesized from two simple precursors, glycine and succinyl coenzyme A.
- Synthesis of heme begins in the mitochondria and ends in the mitochondria, with some intermediate steps occurring in the cytosol.
- ALA synthase is the rate-limiting enzyme of hepatic biosynthesis of heme.

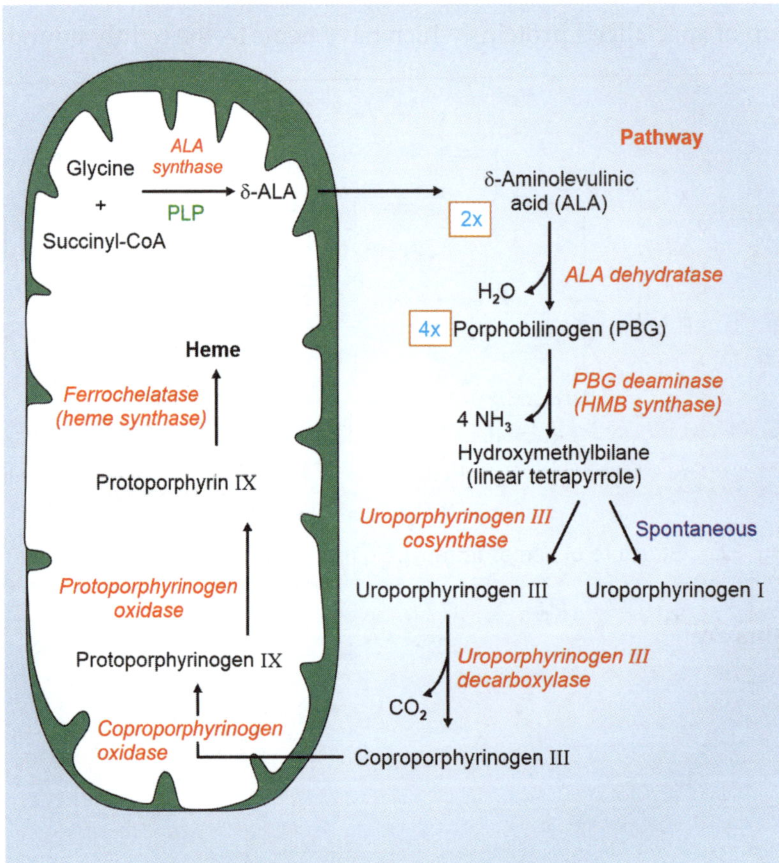

Fig. 32.2: Heme synthesis

Key Notes

Heme Degradation/Catabolism

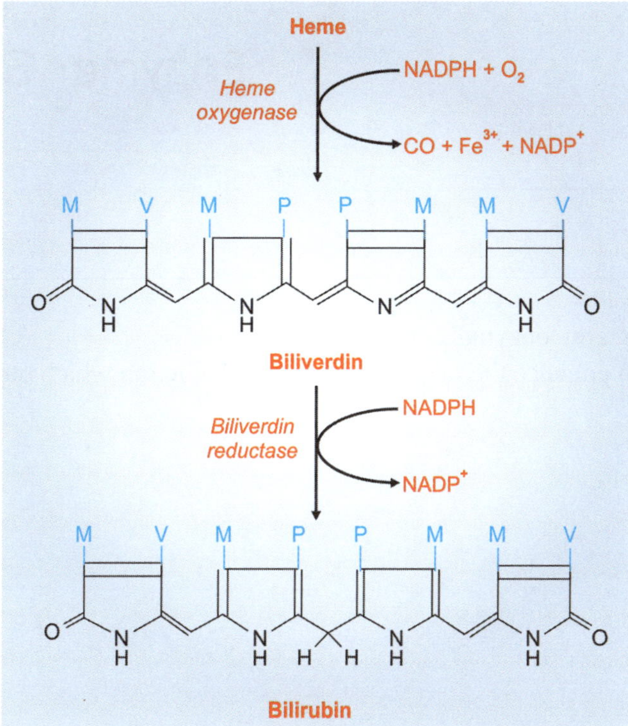

Fig. 32.3: Heme catabolism (note the open tetrapyrrole ring structure of biliverdin and bilirubin)

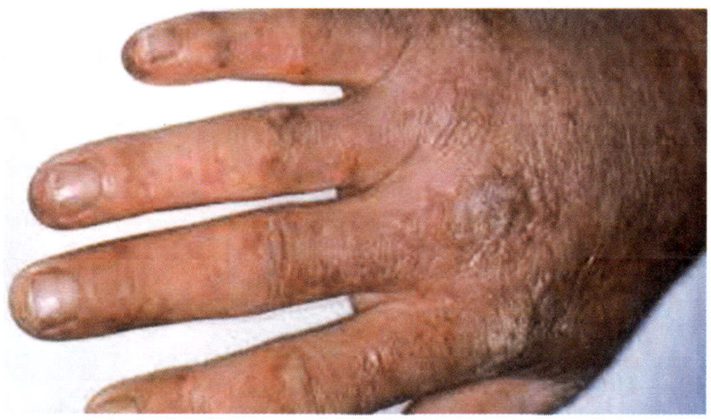

Fig. 32.4: Porphyria—cutaneous manifestation

Key Notes

Section I
Enzyme

33

Enzyme: General Aspects

Key concepts

Friedrich W. Kühne coined the term 'enzyme'.

Enzymes are biocatalysts which enhance the rate of a biochemical reaction which otherwise progresses very slowly in absence of enzyme.

Classification of enzymes

Six major classes:

I. Oxidoreductase
II. Transferase
III. Hydrolase
IV. Lyase
V. Isomerase
VI. Ligase

Mode of action of enzyme

Enzymes act via lowering the 'activation energy'

Activation Energy Lowering to the Presence of Enzyme

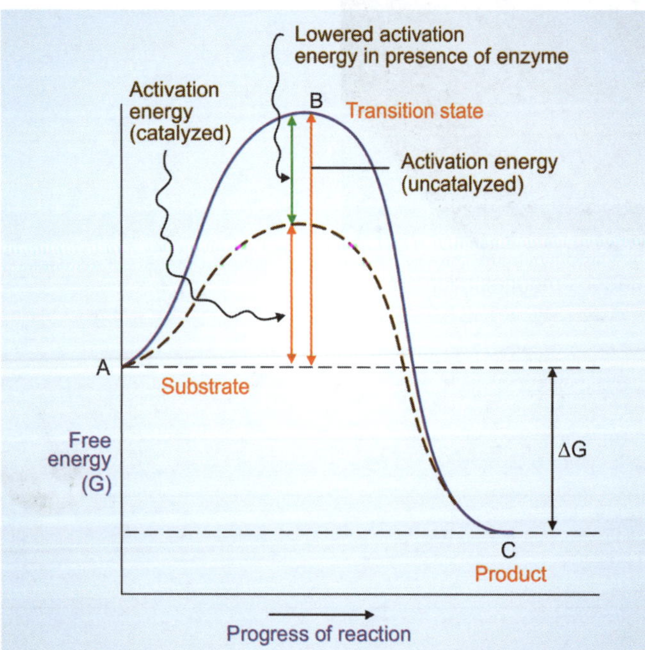

Fig. 33.1: Lowering of activation energy by enzyme

Key Notes

> ***Key concepts***
> ***Models to explain the binding of substrate to the active site of the enzyme***
> - Lock and key model (rigid template model): By Emil Fischer (1894)
> - Induced fit model (hand in glove model): By Daniel E. Koshland (1958)

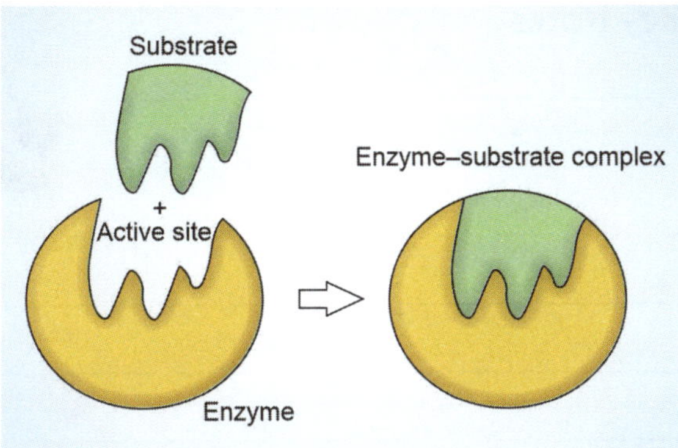

Fig. 33.2: Lock and key model (Emil Fischer, 1894)

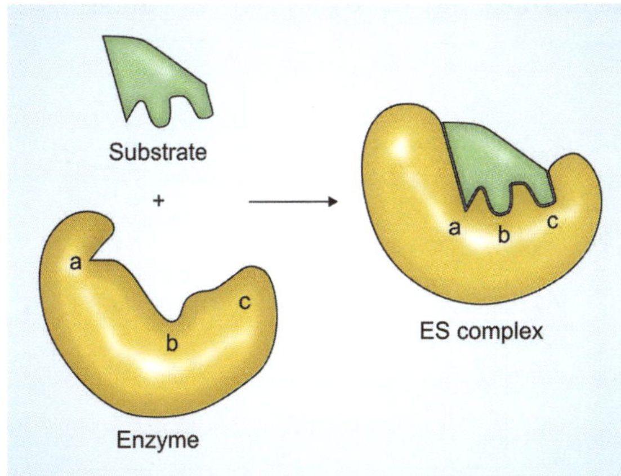

Fig. 33.3: Induced fit model (Daniel E. Koshland, 1958)

> ***Key concepts***
> *Factors which affect the enzyme kinetics are:*
> 1. Substrate concentration
> 2. Temperature
> 3. pH
> 4. Enzyme concentration
> 5. Product concentration
> 6. Inhibitors

Effect of Substrate Concentration on Enzyme Kinetics

The reaction velocity progressively increases with substrate concentration until the maximum velocity is reached at one specific substrate concentration.

Beyond this, the rate of reaction does not increase as all the active site of the enzyme is saturated with substrate, and a further increase in substrate concentration does not increase the reaction rate.

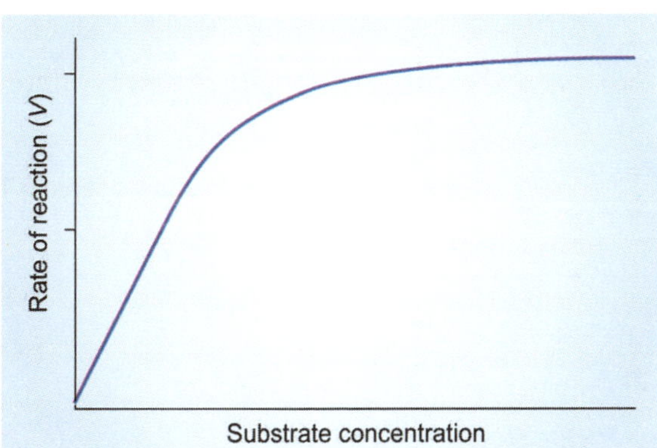

Fig. 33.4: Effect of substrate concentration on reaction velocity

Key Notes

Michaelis-Menten Constant (K_m)

- It is defined as the substrate concentration required to achieve half of V_{max}.
- K_m value has the unit which is the same as substrate concentration.
- K_m value is specific for the enzyme and its corresponding substrate.
- K_m value is inversely proportional to the affinity of the enzyme and its substrate.
- Isoenzymes may have different K_m values.

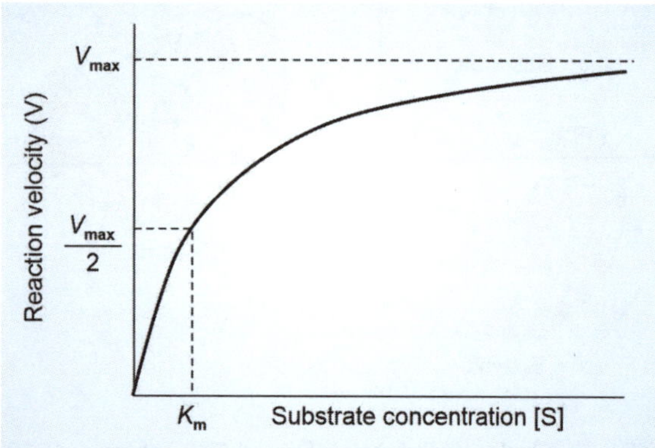

Fig. 33.5: Plot to show K_m value (Michaelis-Menten constant)

Key Notes

Effect of Temperature on Enzyme Kinetics (Bell-shaped Curve)

At optimum temperature, the enzyme acts maximally, and the enzyme activity is compromised on either side of optimum temperature.

Key Notes

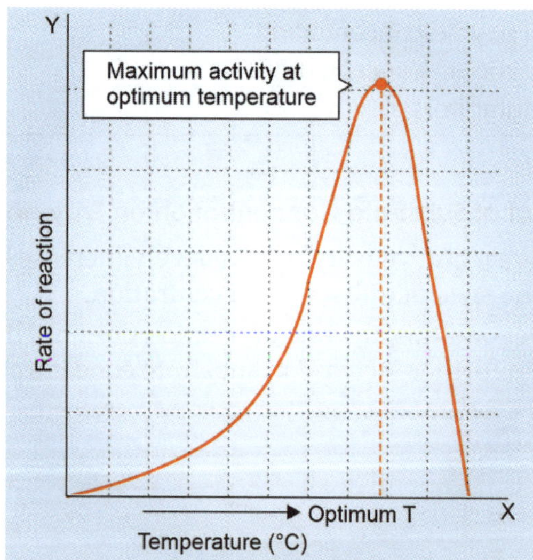

Fig. 33.6: Bell-shaped curve to show optimum T

Effect of H^+ Concentration (pH) on Enzyme Kinetics

- Even for pH, the enzyme kinetic shows a bell-shaped curve.
- At optimum pH, the enzyme acts maximally, and on either side of optimum pH the enzyme activity is compromised.

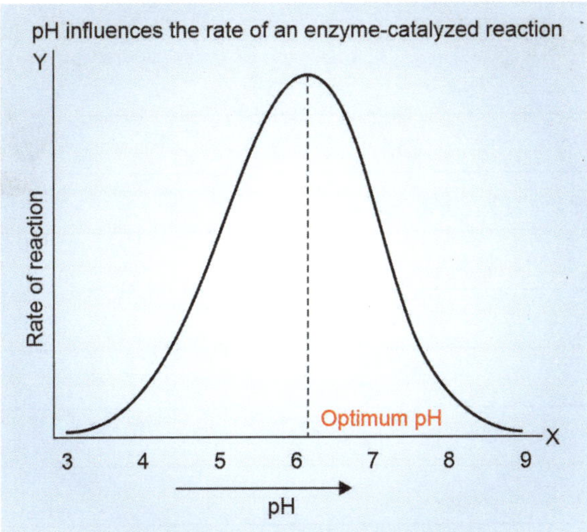

Fig. 33.7: Bell-shaped curve to show optimum pH

Key Notes

Effect of Enzyme Concentration on Enzyme Kinetics

The impact of enzyme concentration on enzyme kinetics shows a linear graph, which means the rate of reaction increases with an increase in enzyme concentration. This is due to the availability of more of the active site with increasing enzyme concentration for the reaction to proceed, increasing the reaction rate.

Key Notes

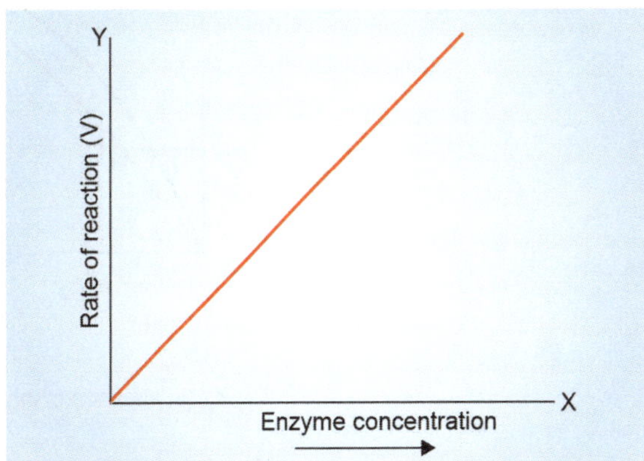

Fig. 33.8: Effect of enzyme concentration on reaction velocity

Special note

- Lineweaver-Burk plot (double reciprocal plot).
- In this plot reciprocal values of substrate concentration and velocity is plotted on X and Y axis respectively.
- In this plot the enzyme kinetic gives linear line which intercepts the Y axis at $1/V_{max}$ point.

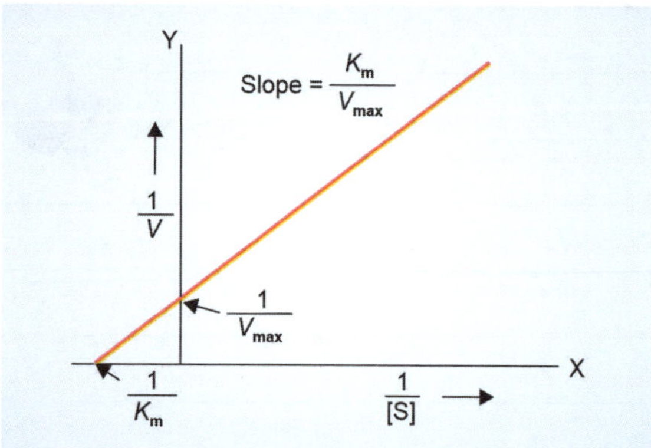

Fig. 33.9: Lineweaver-Burk plot (double reciprocal plot)

Key Notes

Effect of Inhibitors on Enzyme Kinetics

a. Competitive inhibitors do not alter the velocity maximum value but increase the K_m value.

b. Non-competitive inhibitors reduce the value of V_{max} but do not change the K_m value for new lowered velocity.

c. Uncompetitive inhibitors reduce both V_{max} and K_m value.

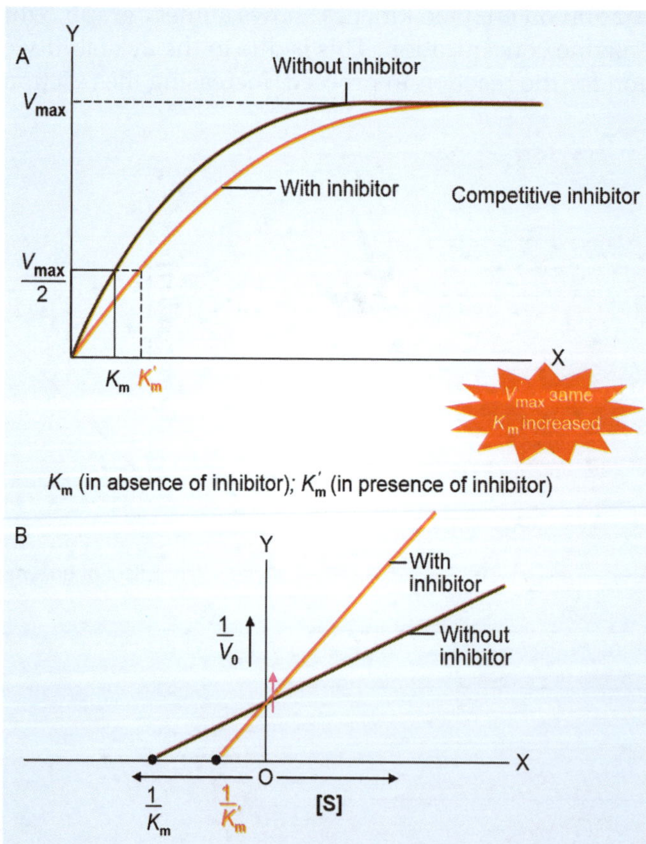

Fig. 33.10: Effect of competitive inhibitors (A = effect shown on Michaelis-Menten plot, B = effect shown on Lineweaver-Burk plot)

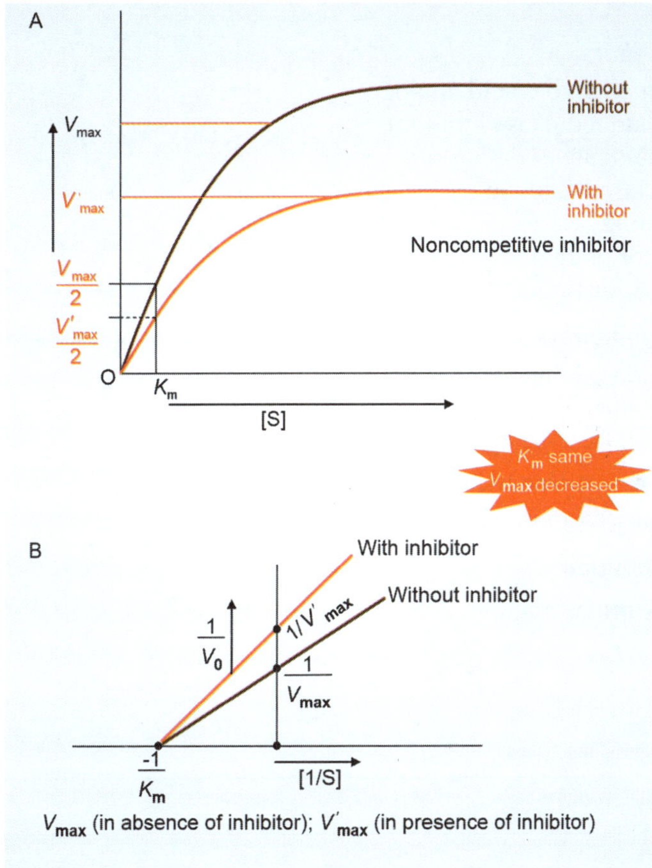

Fig. 33.11: Effect of noncompetitive inhibitors (A = effect shown on Michaelis-Menten plot; B = effect shown on Lineweaver-Burk plot)

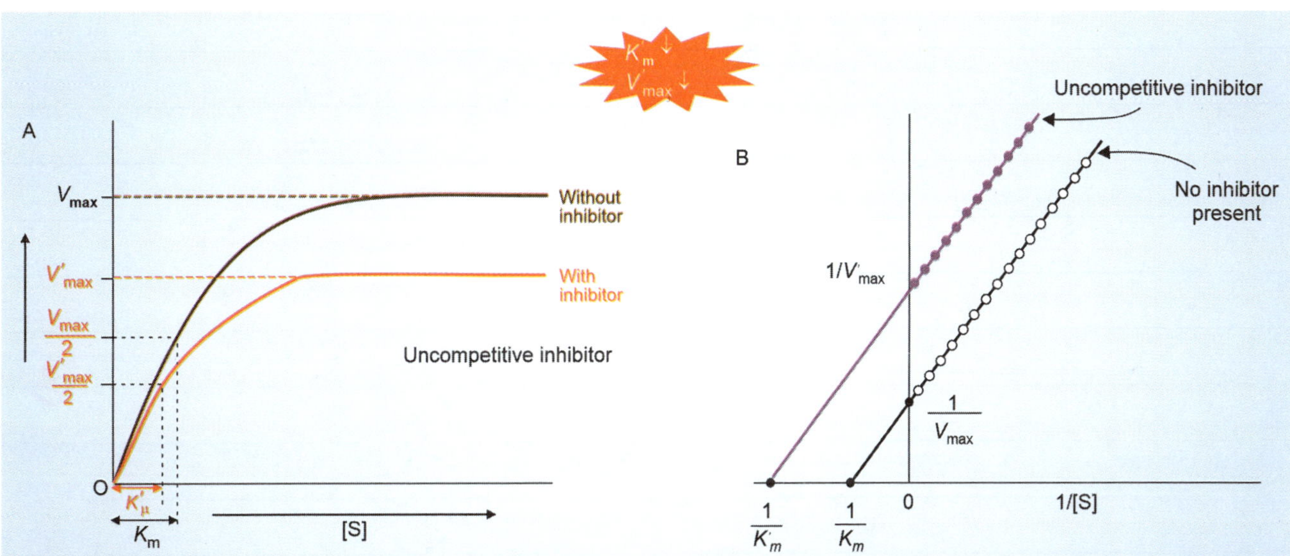

Fig. 33.12: Effect of uncompetitive inhibitors (A = effect shown on Michaelis-Menten plot; B = effect shown on Lineweaver-Burk plot)

Clinical Correlation

Examples of competitive inhibitors

1. Sulphonamide as para-aminobenzoic acid analogue
2. Methotrexate as dihydrofolate reductase inhibitor
3. Dicumarol as vitamin K analogue
4. Statins as HMG-CoA reductase analogue
5. Ethanol in methanol poisoning
6. 5-Fluorouracil as an inhibitor of thymidylate synthase
7. Isoniazid (INH) as vitamin B_6 analogue

Examples of noncompetitive inhibitors

1. Cyanide as cytochrome oxidase inhibitor
2. Fluoride as enolase inhibitor in glycolysis
3. Iodoacetate as inhibitor of glyceraldehyde-3-phosphate dehydrogenase
4. British-Anti-Lewisite (BAL) as antidote of heavy metal poisoning
5. Organophosphorus poisoning as an inhibitor of acetylcholinesterase.

Example of uncompetitive inhibition

Inhibition of placental ALP by phenylalanine.

Key Notes

Metallic Cofactors for Specific Enzyme

Table 33.1: Inorganic elements as a cofactor for certain enzymes

Element	Enzymes
Copper (Cu^{2+})	• Superoxide dismutase (SOD) • Monoamine oxidase (MAO) • Lysyl oxidase • Cytochrome oxidase • ALA synthase • Tyrosinase
Iron (Fe^{2+}/Fe^{3+})	• Cytochrome oxidase • Catalase • Peroxidase • Proline hydroxylase
Potassium (K^{+})	• Pyruvate kinase
Magnesium (Mg^{2+})	• Hexokinase • Glucose-6-phosphatase • Pyruvate kinase
Manganese (Mn^{2+})	• Arginase • Superoxide dismutase (SOD) • Ribonucleotide reductase
Selenium (Se)	• Glutathione peroxidase (GPO) • Deiodinase
Zinc (Zn^{2+})	• Carbonic anhydrase • Alcohol dehydrogenase • Carboxypeptidase A and B • ALA synthase • Superoxide dismutase (SOD) • RNA polymerase • ALP • LDH
Molybdenum (Mo)	• Xanthine oxidase • Sulphite oxidase • Aldehyde oxidase • Dinitrogenase
Ni	• Urease

Table 33.2: Coenzymes and the group they transfer

Coenzyme	*Group they transfer*	*Dietary precursor*
Biocytin	CO_2	Biotin
Coenzyme A	Acyl group	Pantothenic acid and other compounds
FAD	Electron	Riboflavin (vitamin B_2)
Lipoate	Electron and acyl group	Not required in diet
NAD	Hydride ion (H^-)	Nicotinic acid (niacin)
Pyridoxal phosphate (PLP)	Amino group	Pyridoxine (B_6)
Tetrahydrofolic acid (THF)	1 carbon group	Folate
Thiamine pyrophosphate (TPP)	Aldehyde	Thiamine
Coenzyme B_{12} (5′-deoxyadenosylcobalamin)	H atom and alkyl group	Vitamin B_{12}

34 Clinical Enzymology

ENZYME AS A MARKER IN MYOCARDIAL INFARCTION

Table 34.1: Enzymes in assessment of myocardial infarction (time of appearance, peak level and decline)

Enzymes	Appearance in plasma (post-MI)	Time of peak level	Decline to low level
CPK (MB)	4–8 hours	1 day (24 hours)	2–3 days
AST	24–36 hours	2 days (48 hours)	4–6 days
LDH	8–10 hours	2–3 days	10–15 days

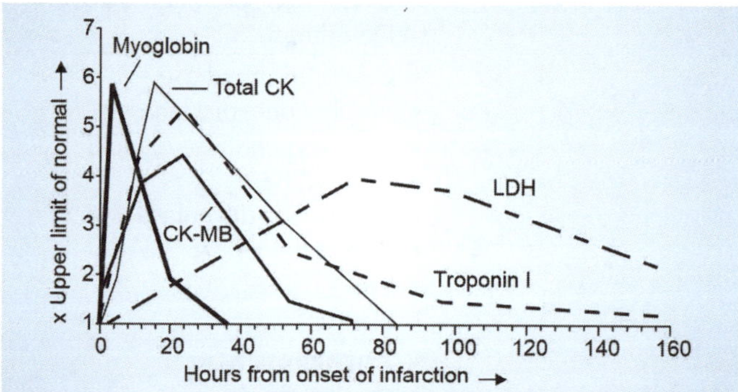

Fig. 34.1: Graph representing the onset, peak and decline of various enzyme markers in a typical case of myocardial infarction

ENZYMES AS A MARKER IN LIVER DISEASE

a. AST (SGOT): Aspartate transaminase
b. ALT (SGPT): Alanine transaminase
c. ALP: Alkaline phosphatase
d. GGT: Gamma-glutamyltransferase

Key Notes

Enzymes as a Marker in Pancreatic Disease

Serum Amylase

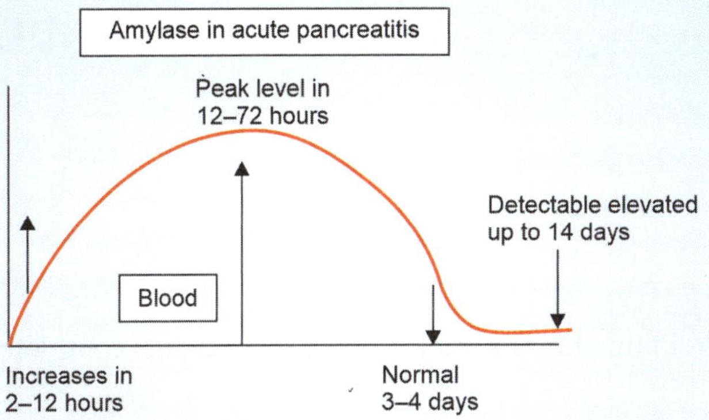

Serum amylase: Timeline of onset of increase, peak and decline in a case of acute pancreatitis

Timeline	Amylase	Lipase
Onset	2–12 hours	4–8 hours
Peak	12–72 hours	24 hours
Decline	3–4 days	8–14 days

Serum Lipase

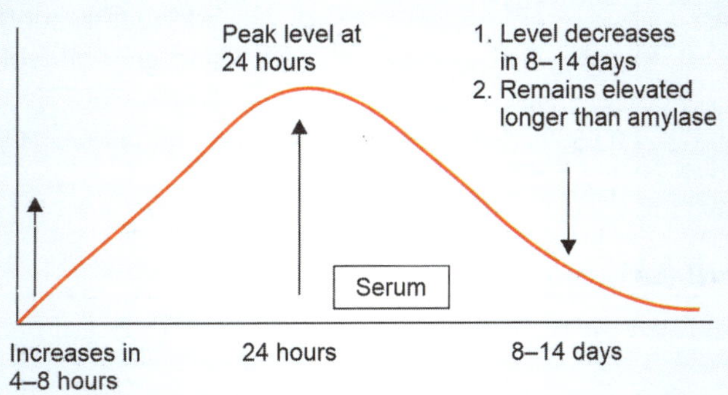

Serum lipase: Timeline of onset of increase, peak and decline in a case of acute pancreatitis

Key Notes

35 Nutrition

CALORIFIC VALUE OF VARIOUS FOOD ITEMS

Calorific value is defined as the "Amount of heat energy obtained by burning 1.0 gm of foodstuff completely in the presence of oxygen".

Table 35.1: Calorific value, RQ, SDA of various food items

Nutrient	Calorific value	RQ	SDA
Carbohydrate	4 kcal/gm	1.0	5%
Protein	4.2 kcal/gm	0.84	30%
Lipid	9 kcal/gm	0.71	15%
Mixed diet	—	0.85	10%
Alcohol	7 kcal/gm	0.66	—

Balanced Diet

A balanced diet is defined as one which contains a variety of foods in such quantity and proportion that need for energy and all nutrients are adequately met for maintaining health, vitality and general well-being

ESTIMATED AVERAGE REQUIREMENT (EAR)

Amount of nutrient estimated to meet the nutrient requirement of half (50%) of healthy individuals in an age and gender group.

RECOMMENDED DIETARY ALLOWANCE (RDA)

Amount of nutrient estimated to meet the nutrient requirement of 97–98% of healthy individual population RDA = (EAR + 2 SD).

BASAL METABOLIC RATE (BMR)

- It is minimal energy required by the body to sustain life and maintain vital functions of the body.
- It is defined as 'energy expenditure by the body when at rest (physical, emotional and digestive) but not asleep, under thermal neutrality (at 25°C), estimated after 12 hours of 'fasting'.

Normal Value of BMR

- Adult male: 35 kcal/m^2/hour
- Adult female: 32 kcal/m^2/hour.

SPECIFIC DYNAMIC ACTION (SDA) OR DIET-INDUCED THERMOGENESIS

- This is the energy utilized in the processing of food like digestion, absorption, active transport, etc.
- Proteins have the greatest SDA, about 30% above their caloric value.
- Carbohydrates and lipids have SDA of 5% and 15%, respectively.
- For a mixed diet, SDA may be calculated as 10%.

RESPIRATORY QUOTIENT (RQ)

- RQ is 'ratio of volume of CO_2 produced by a volume of O_2 consumed during a given time by utilizing one gram.
- RQ = Volume of CO_2 produced/volume of O_2 consumed.
  a. RQ of the carbohydrate is 1.
  b. RQ of the protein is 0.84.
  c. RQ of the fat is 0.71.
  d. RQ of mixed diet is about 0.85.

NUTRITIONAL INDICES OF PROTEIN

1. **Biological value (BV) of protein:** This is the ratio of nitrogen retained and nitrogen absorbed during a specific interval.
   BV = Nitrogen retained/nitrogen absorbed × 100
2. **Net protein utilization (NPU):** Ratio of nitrogen retained to that of the nitrogen intake multiplied by 100.
   NPU = Nitrogen retained/nitrogen intake × 100
   NPU is better marker of protein quality than BV.

GLYCEMIC INDEX

It is defined as "Effect of 50 gm of carbohydrate in a particular food item on blood glucose level compare to 50 gm of pure anhydrous glucose".

LIMITING AMINO ACID

Amino acid, deficient in a protein, is known as a limiting amino acid.

- Methionine is the limiting amino acid in the pulses.
- Lysine is a limiting amino acid in the cereals.

NITROGEN BALANCE

When daily dietary nitrogen intake (calculated as 16% of protein intake) is equal to daily nitrogen lost collectively through urine, faeces and sweat, it is called a state of nitrogen balance.

Factors which Lead to Positive Nitrogen Balance

a. Period of growth
b. Pregnancy
c. Lactation
d. Convalescence
e. Anabolic hormones like insulin, growth hormone and androgens.

Factors which Lead to Negative Nitrogen Balance

a. Acute illness: Surgery, trauma and burn
b. Chronic disease: Malignancy and uncontrolled diabetes mellitus
c. Protein deficiency in malnutrition
d. Starvation

PROTEIN-ENERGY MALNUTRITION (PEM)

Marasmus

Marasmus is due to continuous deficiency of both dietary energy and protein.

- No edema
- Thin skin
- Frequent diarrhea
- Weight loss of the baby
- Face shrunken
- Good appetite

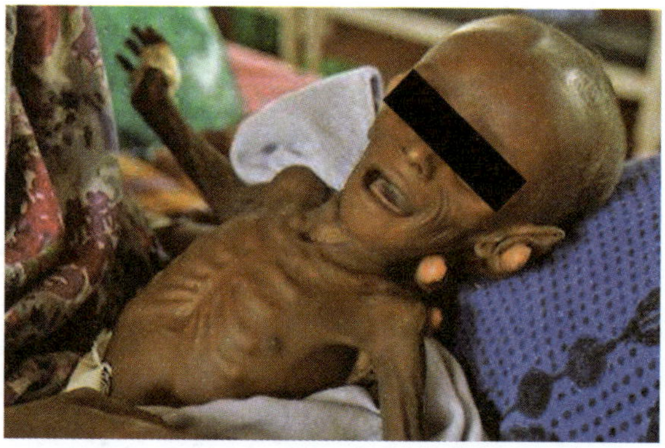

Fig. 35.1: Marasmus child

Kwashiorkor

- Kwashiorkor is due to isolated deficiency of protein alone and adequate calorie supply.
- Generalized edema is a characteristic sign which is due to hypoalbuminemia.
- Puffy face
- Abdomen protuberant
- Poor appetite

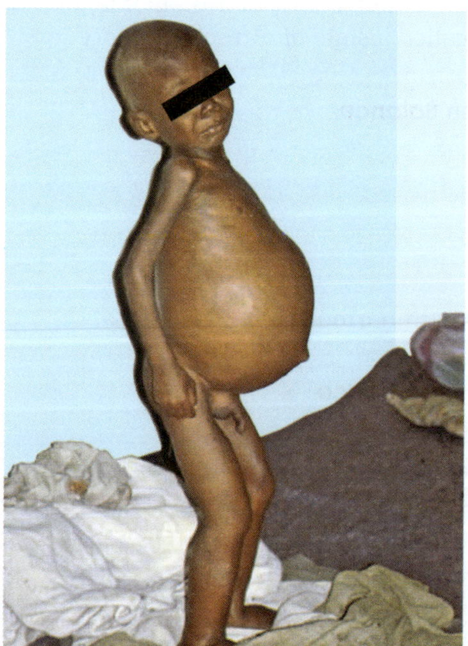

Fig. 35.2: Kwashiorkor (protuberant abdomen and puffy face to note)

Key Notes

36

Vitamins

WATER-SOLUBLE VITAMINS

- Vitamin B_1 is also known as thiamine or anti-beriberi factor or antineuritic vitamin.
- Structure of thiamine consists of a substituted pyrimidine ring (2,5-dimethyl-6-aminopyrimidine) joined to substituted thiazole (4-methyl-5-hydroxyethyl thiazole) via methylene bridge.

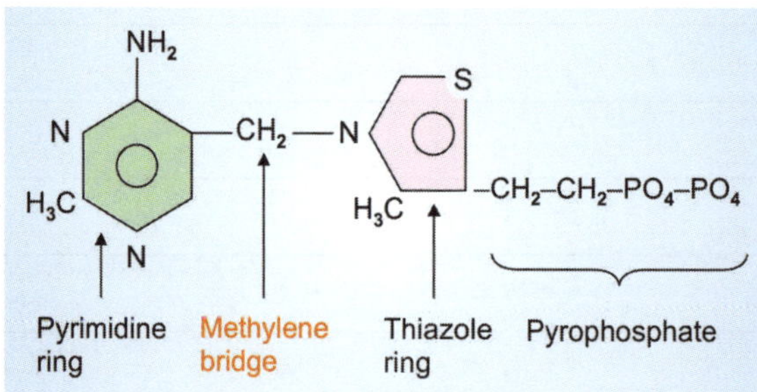

Fig. 36.1: Vitamin B_1 (thiamine) [TPP]

RDA

Adult: 1.0–1.5 mg/day

Children: 0.7–1.2 mg/day

Pregnancy, lactation, old age, alcoholics: 2.0 mg/day

Dietary Sources

- Aleurone layer of cereals
- Pulses
- Oil seeds
- Nut

Deficiency Manifestation of Vitamin B_1 (Thiamine)

- Dry beriberi
- Wet beriberi
- Infantile beriberi
- Wernicke-Korsakoff syndrome

Key Notes

VITAMIN B_2 (RIBOFLAVIN)

- 'Yellow vitamin of 'Warburg' (heat stable but photolabile)
- Structure of riboflavin has a 'dimethyl isoalloxazine ring to which a ribitol is 'attached' through 'N' atom.

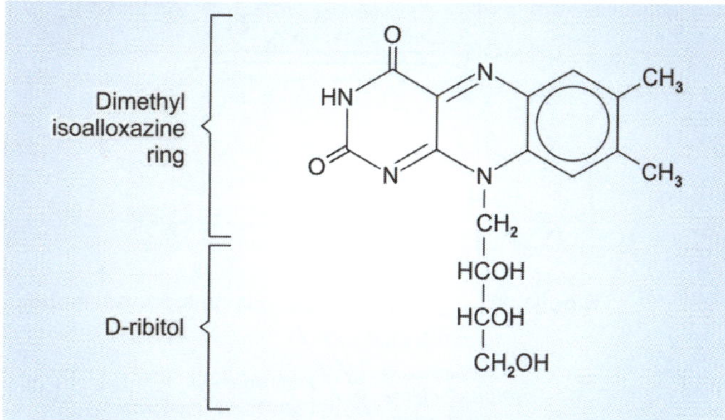

Fig. 36.2: Structure of vitamin B_2 (riboflavin)

Lab Determination

1. RBC glutathione reductase activity (FAD-dependent) can be assessed to assess vitamin B_2 deficiency.
2. Direct assessment of riboflavin in RBC.

Sources

- Liver, dried yeast, egg, whole milk and milk products are rich sources of B_2.
- Fish, whole cereals, legumes, and green leafy vegetables are good sources of B_2.

RDA

Daily requirements 1.5 mg per day. Pregnancy = Additional 0.2 mg [1.5 + 0.2 = 1.7 mg/day]
Lactation = Additional 0.4 mg [1.5 + 0.4 = 1.9 mg/day]

Deficiency

Following are the clinical manifestations of riboflavin deficiency (ariboflavinosis):

- Angular stomatitis
- Cheilosis (dry lips)
- Glossitis (swollen tongue)
- Steatorrhea
- Photophobia
- Circumcorneal vascularization.
- Proliferation of bulbar conjunctival capillaries is the earliest sign of vitamin B_2 deficiency.

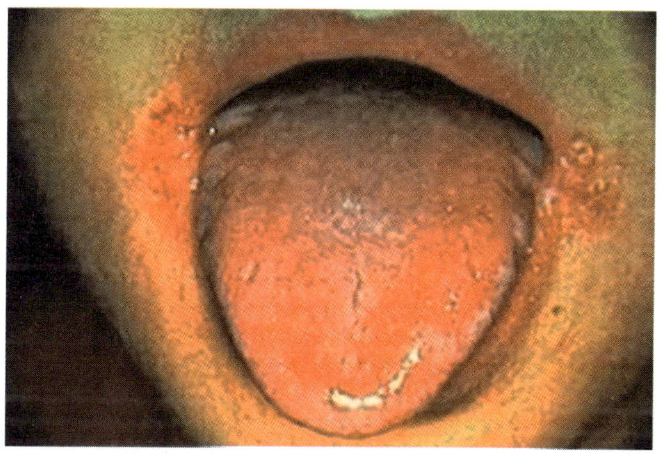

Fig. 36.3: Swollen tongue and cracks at corner of mouth (ariboflavinosis)

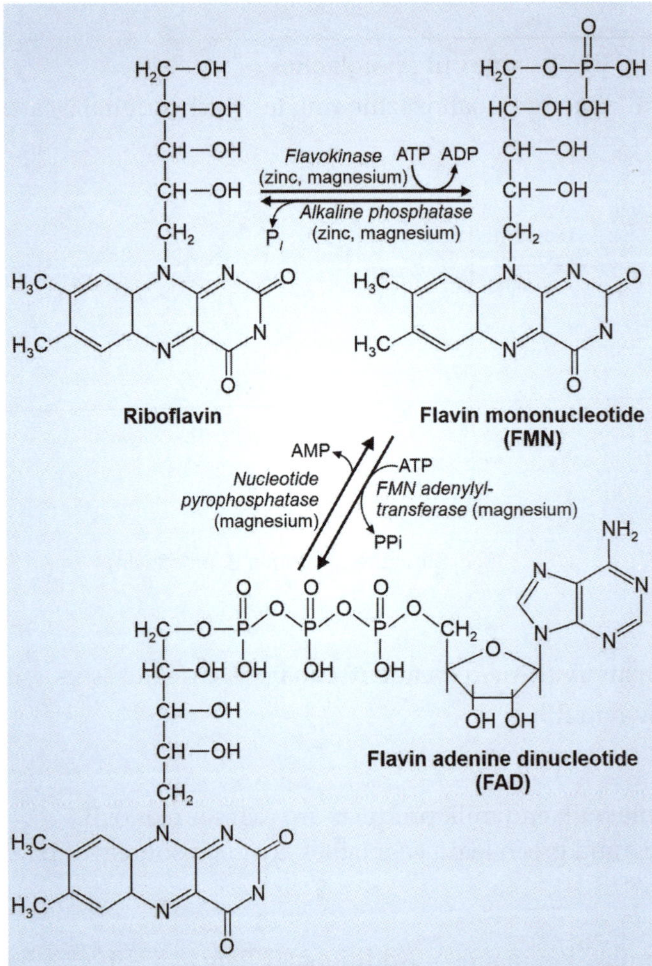

Fig. 36.4: Synthesis of FAD by addition of AMP on FMN

Key Notes

VITAMIN B_3 (NIACIN)

Niacin or nicotinic acid is also known as the 'pellagra preventing factor (PPF) of Goldberger.'

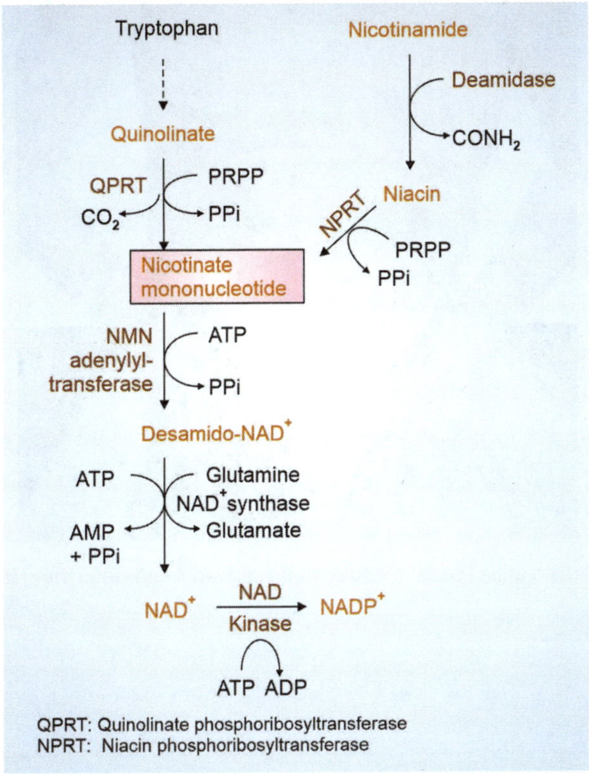

Fig. 36.5: Synthesis of $NAD^+/NADP^+$ from tryptophan in kynurenine pathway

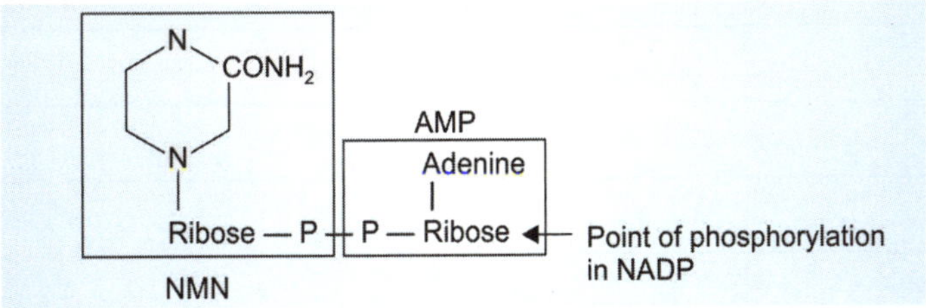

Fig. 36.6: Structure of NAD [NMN + AMP]

RDA

Adult 15–20 mg/day; Child: 10–15 mg/day; Pregnancy: Additional 2 mg/day; Lactation: Additional 5 mg/day

Dietary Sources

Meat, peanuts, legumes, liver, yeast, whole grain, cereals, pulses, fish, egg and vegetables are good sources of vitamin B_3.

Deficiency Symptoms

Deficiency of niacin results in pellagra, a disease is characterized by 4Ds (pellagra—rose skin)

- Diarrhea
- Dermatitis
- Dementia
- Death (in extreme deficiency)

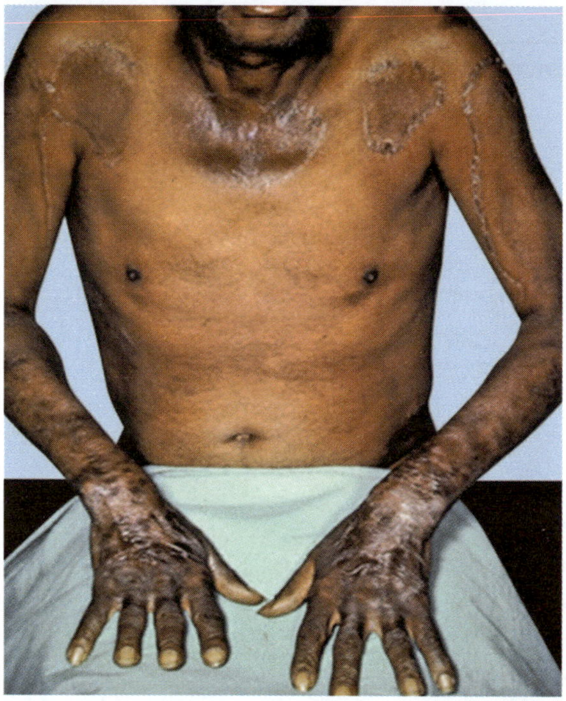

Fig. 36.7: Characteristic of dermatitis (casal necklace and gloved hand deformity) in a typical case of pellagra

Key Notes

VITAMIN B$_5$ (PANTOTHENIC ACID)

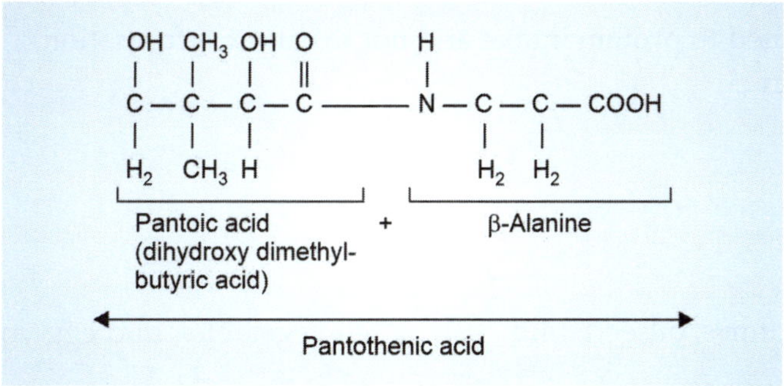

Fig. 36.8: Structure of pantothenic acid (pantoic acid + β-alanine)

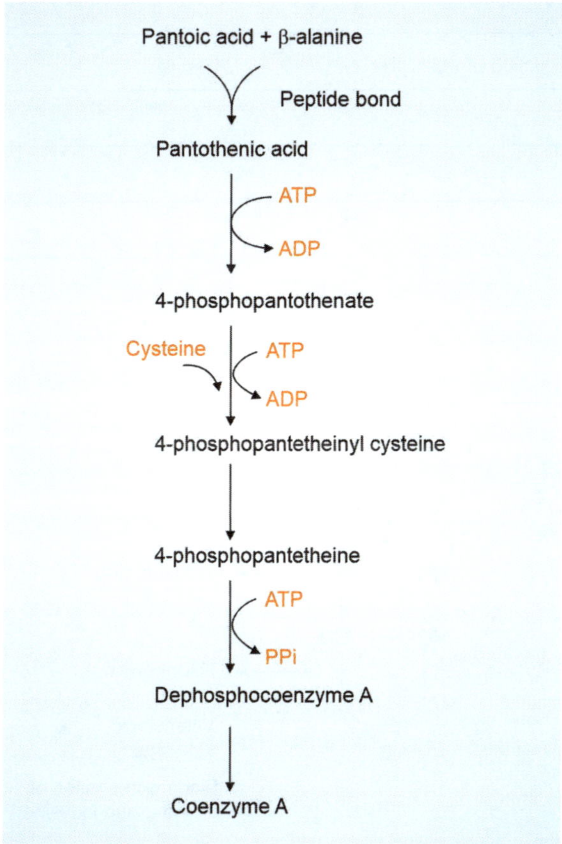

Fig. 36.9: Coenzyme A synthesis from pantothenic acid

RDA

- 5–10 mg/day
- Dietary sources are widely available, so deficiency is rare. The primary sources are egg, liver, meat, yeast, and milk.

VITAMIN B_6

RDA

Vitamin B_6 requirement is related to protein intake and not to caloric information.
Healthy adult: 1.5 to 2.0 mg/day
Pregnancy: 2.5 mg/day
Lactation: 2.5 mg/day
Old age: 2.5 mg/day

Dietary Sources

Meat, whole grain cereals, legumes, oilseed, milk, fish, green vegetables, and egg yolk are rich sources.

Key Notes

VITAMIN B_7 (BIOTIN)

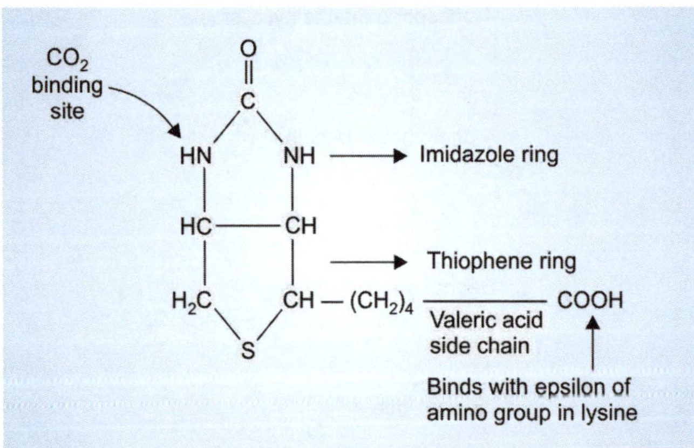

Fig. 36.10: Structure of biotin

RDA

20–30 mg/day

Dietary Sources

- Liver
- Kidney
- Egg yolk
- Milk
- Tomato
- Grain

FOLIC ACID (VITAMIN B_9)

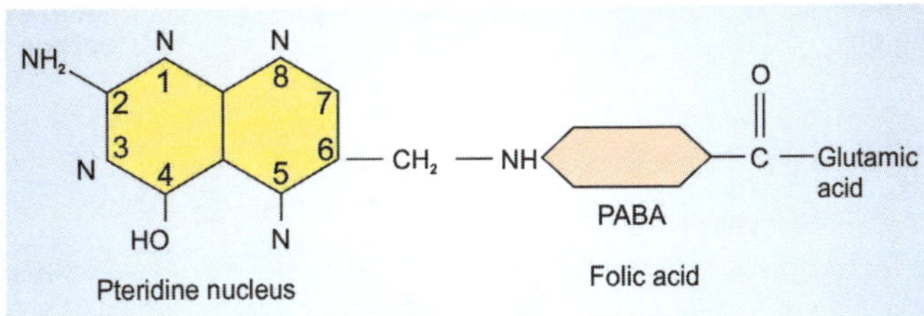

Fig. 36.11: Folic acid composition (pteridine ring + PABA + glutamic acid)

Biochemical Role of Folic Acid

The coenzyme form of folic acid is tetrahydrofolic acid (THF)

Folic acid is involved in one-carbon metabolism and acts as a one-carbon carrier. Various one-carbon moieties which THF transfers are:

1. N5-formyl THF (–CHO)
2. N10-formyl THF (–CHO)
3. N5-formimino THF (–CH = NH)
4. N5N10-methylene THF (= CH_2)
5. N5N10-methenyl THF (–CH)
6. N5-methenyl THF (–CH_3)

RDA

Adult = 200 µg/day

Pregnancy = 400 µg/day

Lactation = 300 µg/day

Dietary Sources

- Green leafy vegetables
- Whole grains
- Cereals
- Liver
- Kidney
- Yeast
- Egg
- Milk

Key Notes

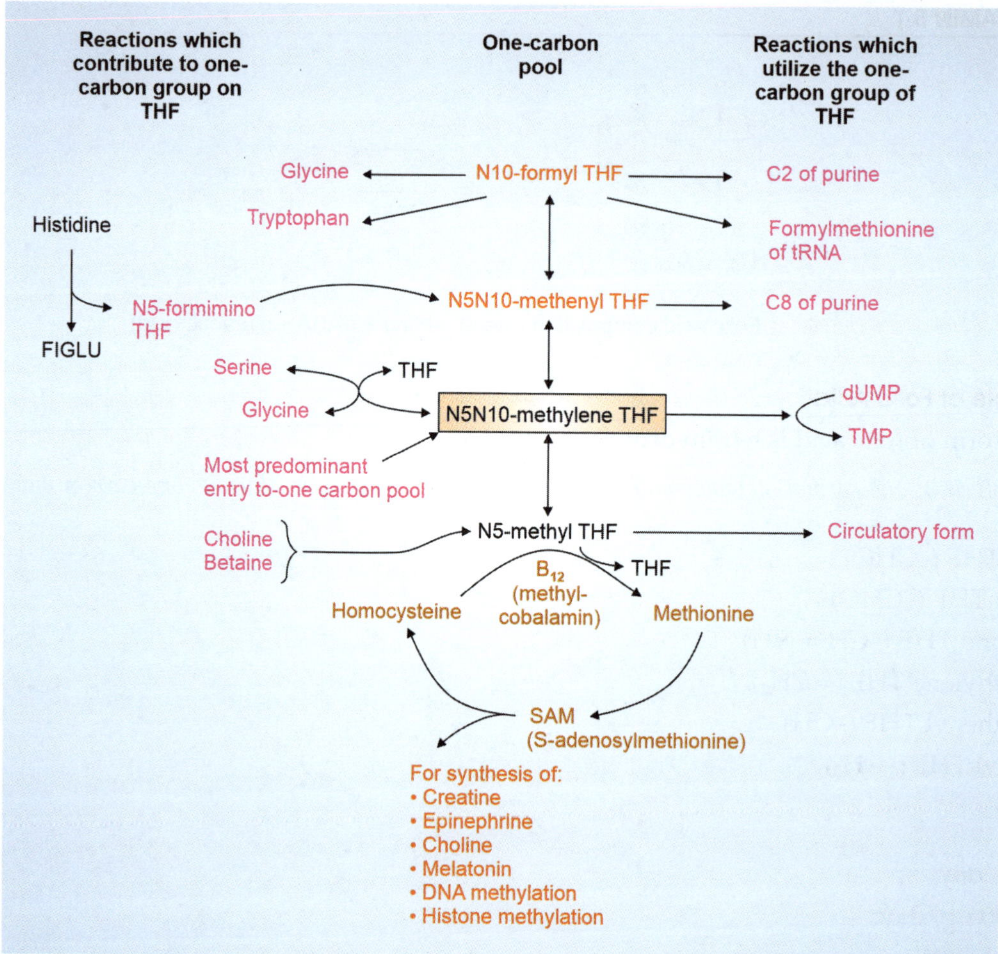

Fig. 36.12: One-carbon metabolism

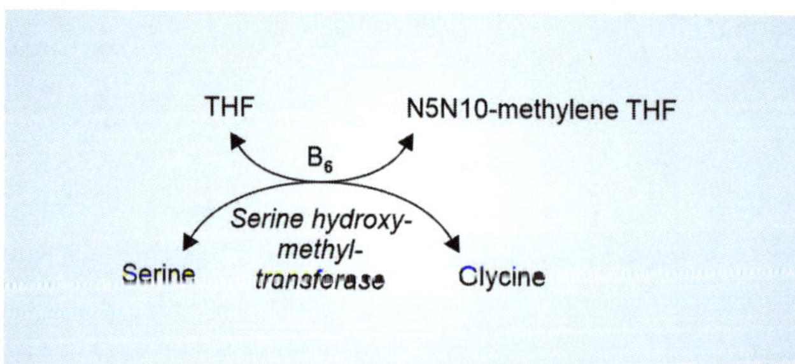

Fig. 36.13: Requirement of free THF for N5N10-methylene THF synthesis

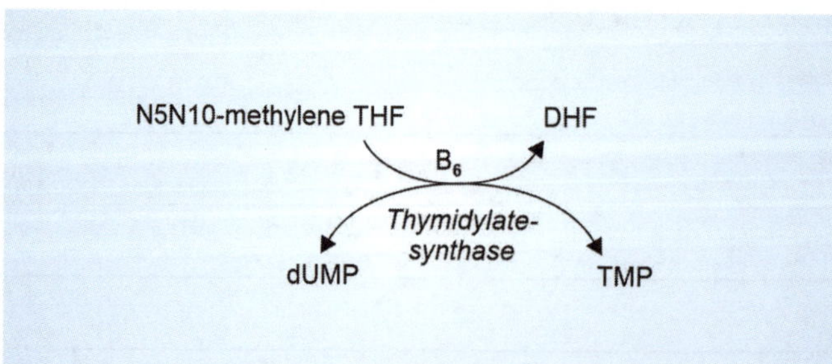

Fig. 36.14: Formation of TMP from dUMP

Key Notes

VITAMIN B_{12}

Vitamin B_{12} is also known as the anti-pernicious anaemia factor or extrinsic factor of Castle (as it needs an intrinsic factor for its intestinal absorption).

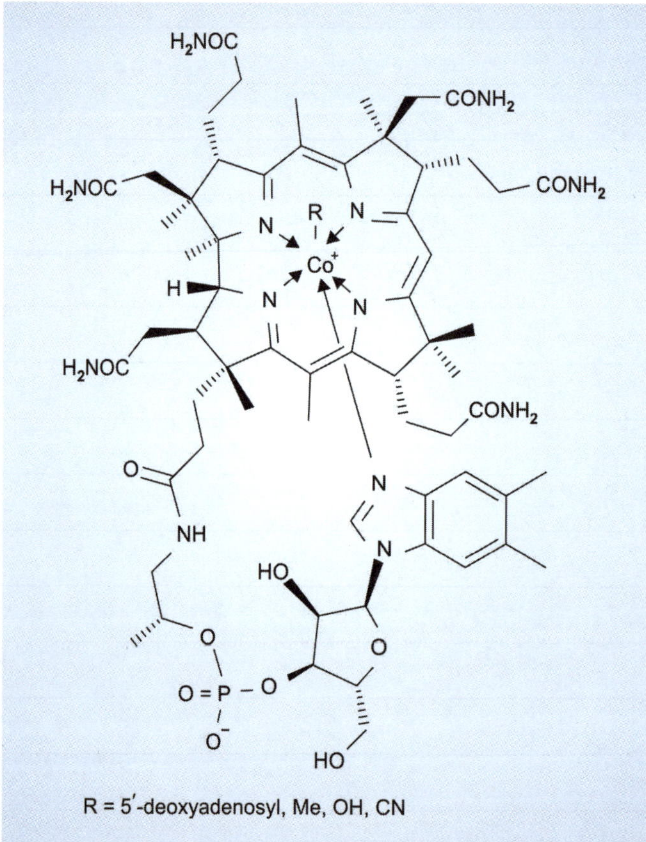

Fig. 36.15: Structure of vitamin B_{12}

Only two human enzymes need vitamin B_{12}. They are:

a. Homocysteine methyl transferase (methionine synthase) and

b. Methyl malonyl-CoA mutase

RDA

- Adult: 1–2 µg/day
- Children: 0.5–1.5 µg/day
- Pregnancy : 3 µg/day
- Lactation : 3 µg/day

Dietary Source

Milk, egg, curd, fish, pork, and chicken are good sources of vitamin B_{12}.

Deficiency Manifestations

1. Megaloblastic anemia
2. Neuronal degeneration and demyelination of the nervous system [subacute combined degeneration (SACD)]
3. Hyperhomocysteinemia

VITAMIN C (ASCORBIC ACID)

- Water soluble
- Heat and alkali labile
- Vitamin C is a potent reducing agent ($Fe^{3+} \rightarrow Fe^{2+}$)
- Reducing property is due to enediol carbon.
- Ascorbic acid is a hexose derivative, closely resembling the structure of monosaccharide.

Biochemical Role

1. Vitamin C is vital for hydroxylation reactions. Following are critical examples where vitamin C plays a role in hydroxylation reactions.

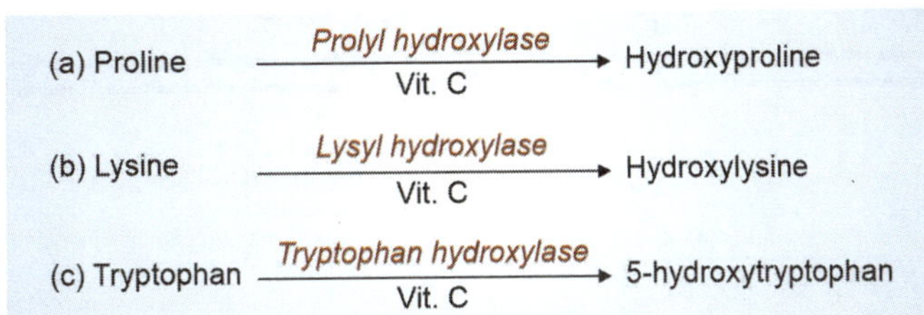

Fig. 36.16: Hydroxylation of proline, lysine and tryptophan by various hydroxylases in vitamin C-dependent manner

2. Vitamin C helps in iron absorption in the gastrointestinal tract lumen. Vitamin C converts Fe^{3+} to Fe^{2+} form, which is then transported across mucosal cell by DMT-1 (divalent metal transporter-1).
3. Methemoglobin is converted to hemoglobin and then to bile pigment in a vitamin C-dependent manner.
4. Vitamin C spares vitamins A, E and specific B complex vitamins by protecting them from oxidation.
5. Activation of folic acid requires vitamin C.
6. Vitamin C acts as an antioxidant vitamin and helps in protection against cataracts, cancer, and cardiovascular disorders.
7. Vitamin C enhances the immunoglolubin synthesis and increases WBC's phagocytic action.
8. Vitamin C is needed for carnitine synthesis, which is important for fatty acid oxidation.
9. RDA 75–90 mg/day for adult nonsmokers and 110–125 mg/day for smokers. Additional 10–20 mg during pregnancy and lactation.

Dietary Sources

- Indian gooseberry (Amla) is the richest source of vitamin C.
- Guava, green vegetables
- Citrus fruits.

Deficiency Symptoms

Following are the deficiency manifestations of vitamin C.

- Capillary fragility
- Decreased wound healing
- Osteoporosis
- Hemorrhages
- Anemia
- Scurvy: Characterized by 'bleeding gums, loose teeth.

FAT-SOLUBLE VITAMINS (VITAMIN D, A, E AND K)

VITAMIN D

Two types of vitamin D are:

i. Vitamin D_2 (ergocalciferol)
ii. Vitamin D_3 (cholecalciferol)

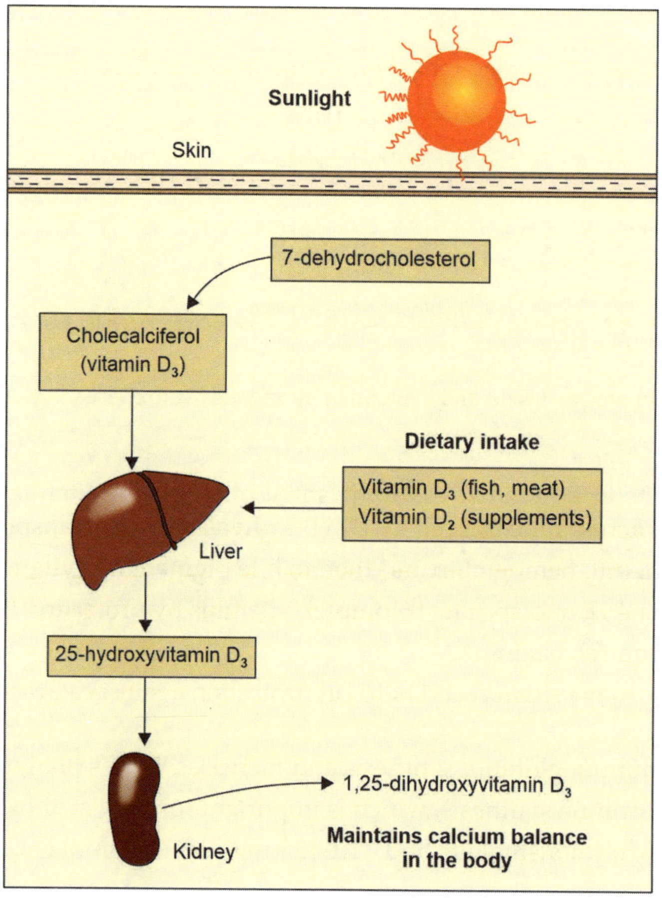

Fig. 36.17: Synthesis of vitamin D in the skin and its activation

Activation of Vitamin D

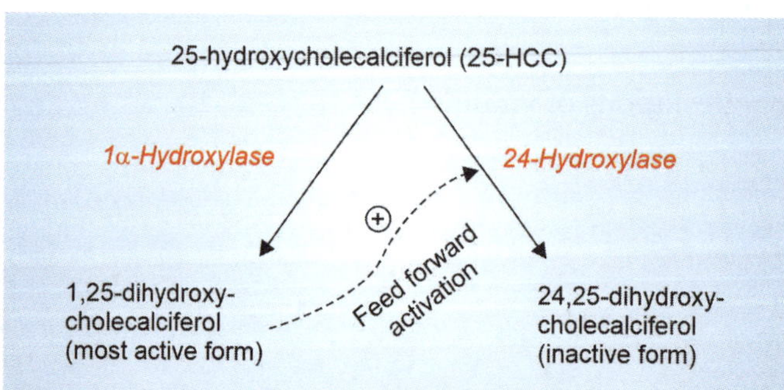

Fig. 36.18: Regulated activation of vitamin D

Effect of Calcitriol on Intestine, Bone and Kidney

- On intestine: 1,25-dihydroxycholecalciferol acts as a typical steroid hormone in gastrointestinal tract mucosa. It induces the synthesis of calbindin, the protein required for calcium transport from the gastrointestinal tract lumen to mucosal cells.
- On bone: 1,25-dihydroxycholecalciferol and PTH synergistically promote bone resorption (demineralization) by stimulating osteoblast formation and activity.
- On kidney (DCT): 1,25-dihydroxycholecalciferol and PTH inhibit calcium excretion via the kidney by stimulating calcium reabsorption at DCT.

RDA: Children: 400 IU/day; Adults: 200 IU/day; Lactation: 400 IU/day (1 mg of cholecalciferol or ergocalciferol = 40 IU)

Sources

- Sunlight
- Fish, egg yolk
- Milk is a poor source.

Deficiency Manifestations

a. Rickets
b. Osteomalacia

Key Notes

VITAMIN A

These compounds are:

1. Retinol
2. Retinal
3. Retinoic acid

RDA

- Adult: 1000 RE in males (3000 IU/day) and 800 RE in females (2500 IU/day)
- 1 IU = 0.3 mg of retinol
- 1 RE = 1 mg of retinol = 12 mg of β-carotene = 24 mg of other carotenoids

Dietary Sources

Liver, kidney, egg yolk, milk, cheese, butter, fish (cod/shark) liver oil-rich sources of vitamin A. Yellow and dark green vegetables and fruits contain carotene.

Deficiency of Vitamin A

1. Night blindness (nyctalopia)
2. Xerophthalmia
3. 'Bitot's spot
4. Keratomalacia (destruction of cornea)
5. Growth retardation
6. Male sterility
7. Rough and dry skin
8. Urinary stone

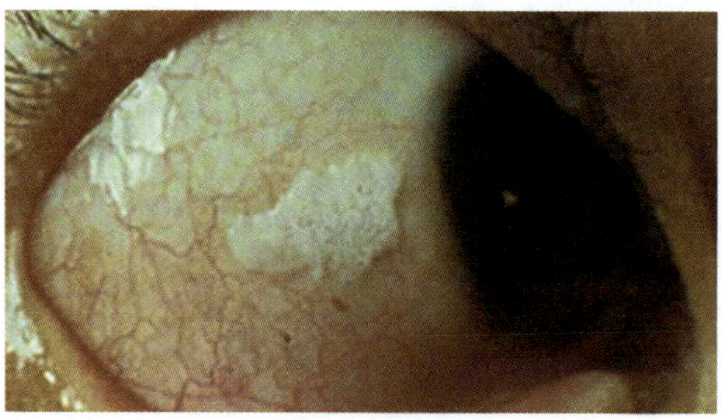

Fig. 36.19: Bitot's spot

Key Notes

VITAMIN E (TOCOPHEROL)

Vitamin E is the most potent biological antioxidant. This is also known as anti-sterility or anti-infertility vitamin.

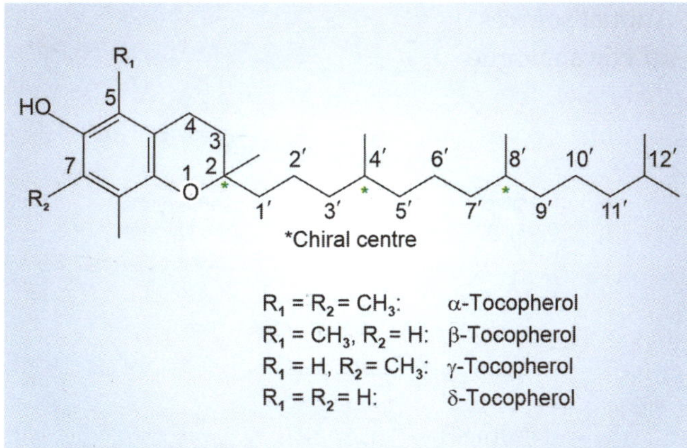

Fig. 36.20: Structure of vitamin E

Vitamin E as an antioxidant.

RDA

- Male = 10 mg of tocopherol (15 IU)
- Female = 8 mg of tocopheorol (12 IU)

Dietary Sources

- Wheat gram oil
- Cotton seed oil
- Peanut oil
- Corn oil
- Sunflower oil

Deficiency Symptoms

- Sterility
- Degenerative changes in muscle
- Megaloblastic anemia
- CNS changes
- Vitamin E is the least toxic amongst fat-soluble vitamins.

Key Notes

VITAMIN K

Three forms of vitamin K are:

1. Vitamin K_1 (phylloquinone): Plant sources
2. Vitamin K_2 (menaquinone): Animal sources
3. Vitamin K_3 (menadione): Synthetic analogue

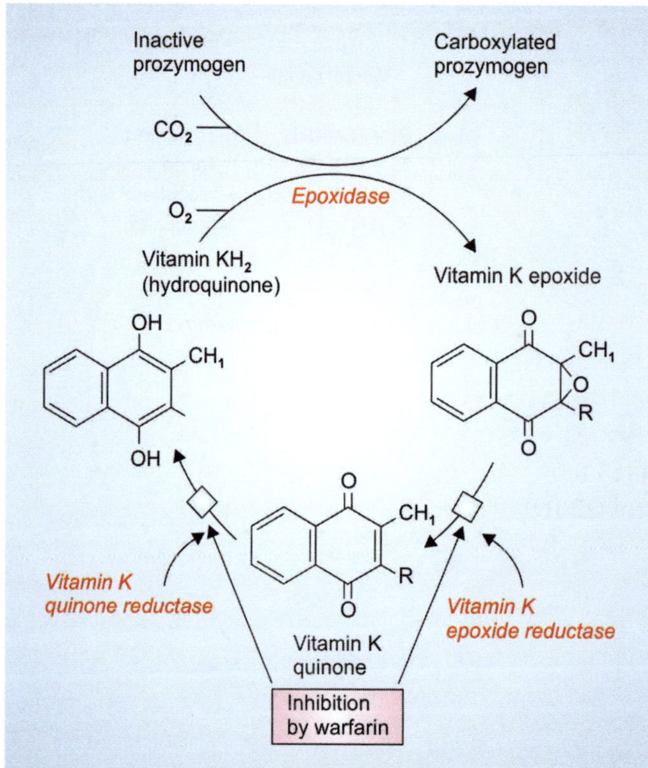

Fig. 36.21: Vitamin K cycle or epoxide cycle

RDA

70–100 mg/day in adults.

Dietary Sources

Good sources of vitamin K are as follows:

- Cabbage
- Cauliflower
- Tomato
- Alfalfa
- Spinach
- Green vegetables

Key Notes

37

Cell and its Organelles

NUCLEUS

- It is the largest organelle of the cell (diameter 10 µm).
- Its main functions are the storage, replication and expression of the genetic material.
- Nucleus is surrounded by an envelop which contains outer and inner nuclear membranes. Inner membrane contains a number of pores of approximately 90Å diameter, and outer membrane is continuous with the rough endoplasmic reticulum and studded with ribosomes (Fig. 37.1).
- Perinuclear space (the space between outer and inner membranes of the nucleus) is continuous with the lumen of rough endoplasmic reticulum.
- In eukaryotic cell, nucleus contains DNA which together with the histone and other structural proteins forms chromatin. During cell divison chromatin further condenses to form chromosome.
- Nucleus is responsible for DNA replication and transcription of various types of RNA.

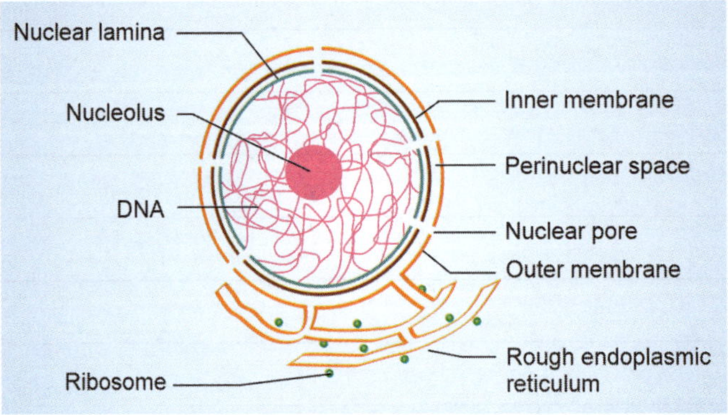

Fig. 37.1: Nucleus

MITOCHONDRIA

- Size of a mitochondrion is about 0.5–1.0 µm in diameter and 7 µm in length. Each cell contains a large number of mitochondria (approx. 2000), which constitute 25% of total cell volume.
- In an electron micrograph, mitochondrion appears as a rod, sphere or filamentous body which is surrounded by an outer and an inner membrane (OMM and IMM).
- Outer membrane is smooth, but inner membrane contains a number of folds or cristae.
- Between outer and inner membranes, there is intermembranous space (Fig. 37.2). Inner membrane is rich in cardiolipin, but has no cholesterol.
- Human mitochondria contain small circular DNA which has code for 2 rRNAs, 22 tRNAs and 13 proteins.
- Outer membrane allows particle less than 10 kDa to pass through it, but inner membrane is completely impermeable, even to small molecules.

- Inner membrane of mitochondria contains numerous transporters, which allow transportation of many metabolites.
- Inner mitochondrial membrane is the host for many enzymes including enzymes of electron transport chain (ETC), which are involved in the process of oxidative phosphorylation.

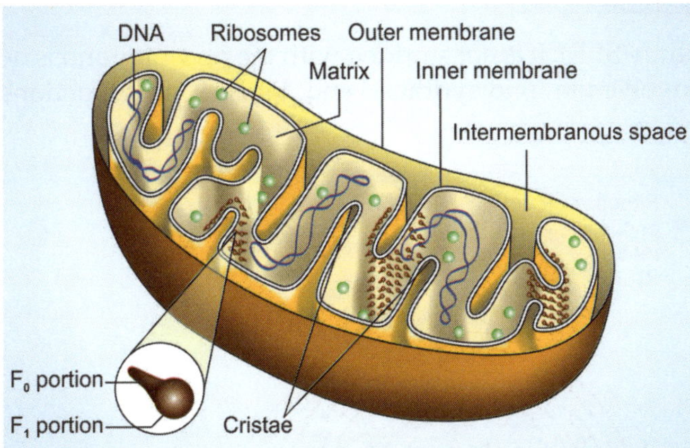

Fig. 37.2: Mitochondrion

Key Notes

Clinical Correlation

- Diseases associated with mutation of mitochondrial DNA
- Leber hereditary optic neuropathy (LHON)
- Myoclonic epilepsy with ragged red fibers (MERRF)
- Mitochondrial encephalopathy, lactic acidosis and stroke-like activity (MELAS)
- Mutation of cytochrome b and exercise intolerance.

ENDOPLASMIC RETICULUM (ER)

- It is a membrane-bound tubular organelle which is continuous with the outer membrane of the nucleus. It is a structure which looks like an interconnected mesh of membrane-bound tubules.
- Rough endoplasmic reticulum (RER): This is the site of protein synthesis. Those proteins which are destined for lysosome, membrane and for export from the cell (secretory proteins) are synthesized in the ribosome of the rough endoplasmic reticulum.
- Smooth endoplasmic reticulum (SER): It is not studded with the ribosome and is not involved in the biosynthesis of the protein, rather, it is involved in lipid synthesis and detoxification reactions.

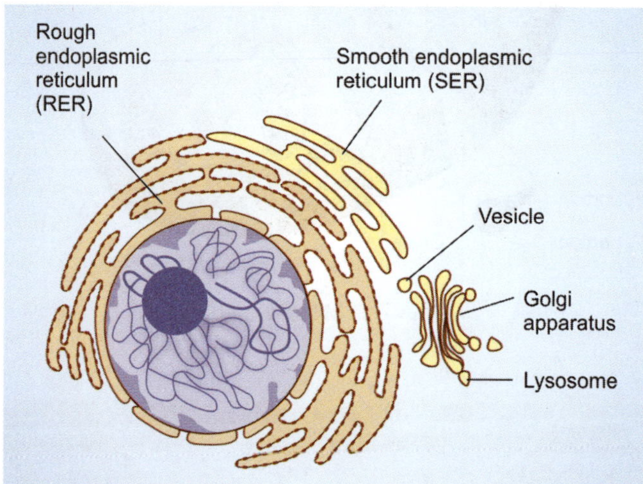

Fig. 37.3: Rough and smooth endoplasmic reticulum

GOLGI APPARATUS

They are involved in the modification and sorting of various proteins, which are to be incorporated into multiple membranes and organelles or have to be secreted out.

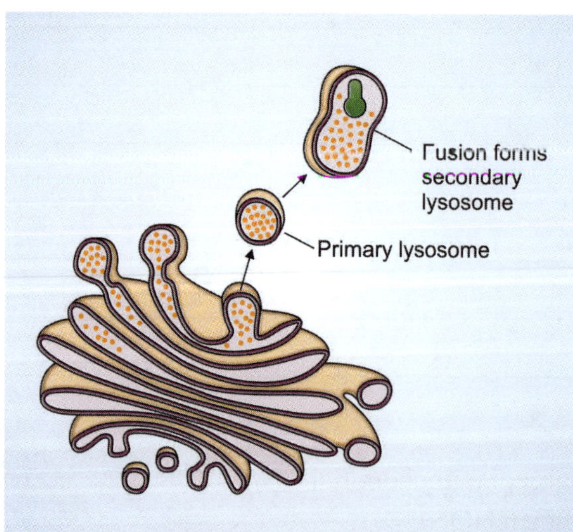

Fig. 37.4: Golgi apparatus

PEROXISOMES

They are also called microbodies (not to be confused with microsome, which is produced due to fragmentation of endoplasmic reticulum during cell fractionation).

As the name implies, these organelles are involved in producing or utilizing hydrogen peroxide. Peroxisomes are spherical and oval in shape and surrounded by a single layer of membrane. Their size is small (0.3–1.5 µm).

They play a significant role in

1. Very long-chain fatty acid (VLCFA) oxidation
2. Synthesis of glycerolipid
3. Synthesis of glycerol-ether lipid (plasmalogen)
4. Synthesis of isoprenoid

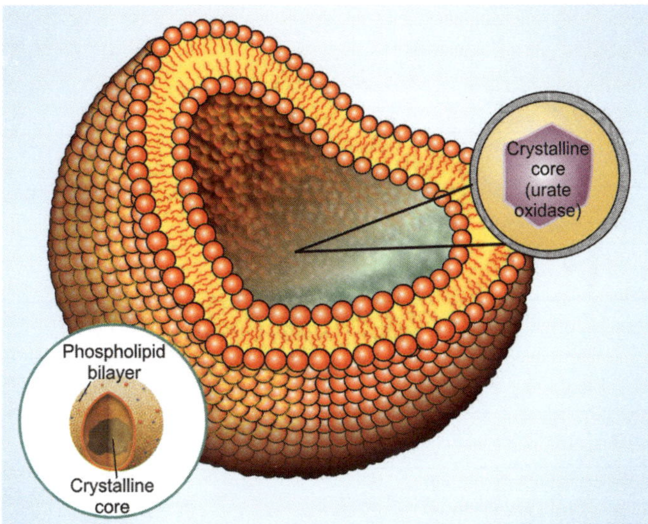

Fig. 37.5: Peroxisome

Key Notes

Lysosomes

- These organelles are rich in the hydrolase class of enzymes (class III), which cleave the carbon–oxygen, carbon–nitrogen, carbon–sulphur, and oxygen–phosphorus bonds in lipids, protein, carbohydrate and nucleic acid.
- The lysosome enzymes act best at acidic pH; intra lysosomal pH is 5.
- Primary lysosome fuses with vesicles containing external material which may have ingested in the cell by phagocytosis, pinocytosis or endocytosis.
- This creates secondary lysosome in the cell, which has both the material and the hydrolase enzyme to digest them.
- Lysosomes are involved in the process called autophagy, whereby they hydrolyze cellular components like proteins, nucleic acids, lipids and organelles like mitochondria.
- I cell disease (inclusion cell disease or mucolipidosis II).

Key Notes

Plasma Membrane

Plasma membrane, also called cell membrane, is the outermost covering of the cell, which separates content of the cell from external environment.

Plasma membrane is made-up of following components

1. Lipids: Phospholipids are the main lipids of membrane. Other lipids in membrane are glycolipids and cholesterol.
2. Proteins in the membrane may be:
   a. Intrinsic (integral)
   b. Extrinsic (peripheral)
3. Carbohydrates

FLUID MOSAIC MODEL OF CELL MEMBRANE (SINGER AND NICOLSON)

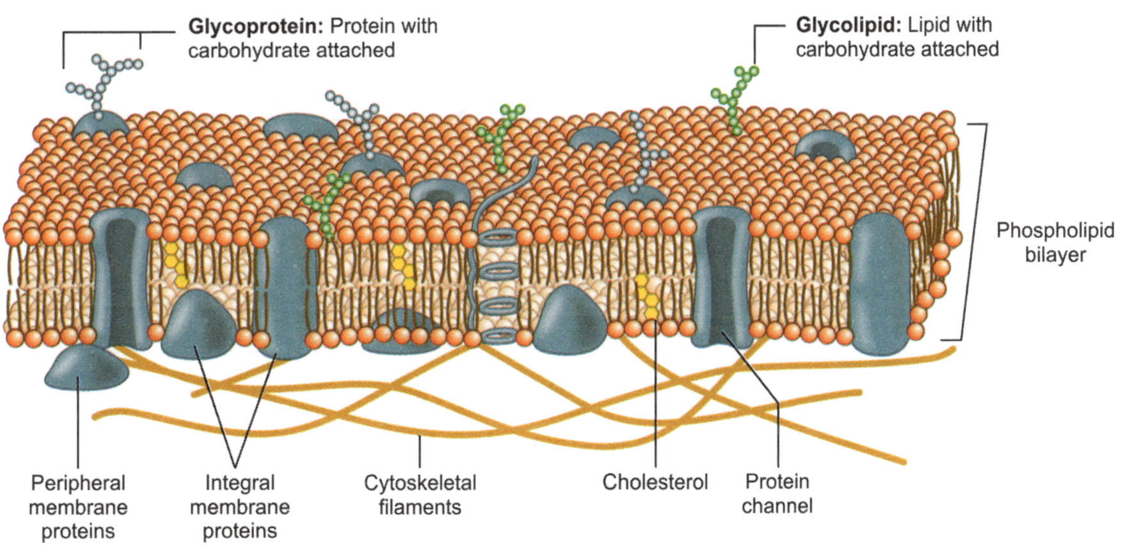

Fig. 38.1: Plasma membrane

Key Notes

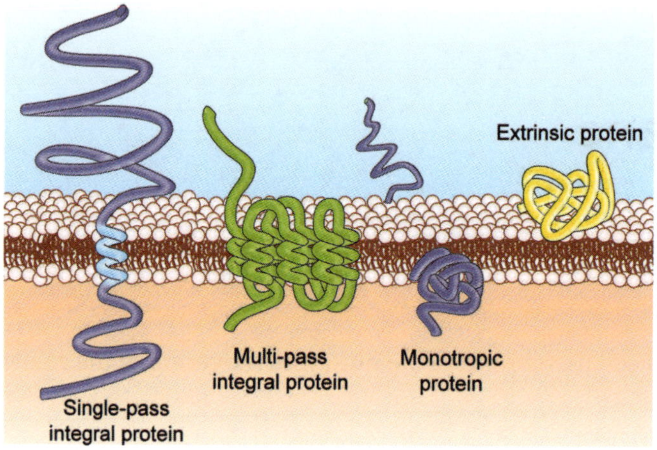

Fig. 38.2: Membrane protein traversing the lipid bilayer

Key Notes

Key Notes

Key Notes

Key Notes

Key Notes

Key Notes

Key Notes

Key Notes

Key Notes